STRET
& FITNESS ROUTINES
FOR EVERYONE

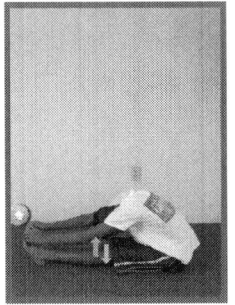

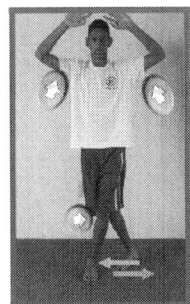

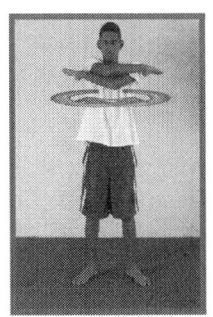

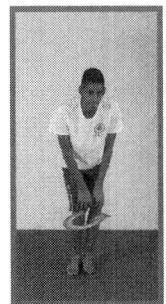

AN EASY GUIDE

TO HEALTH

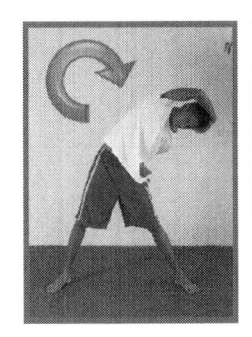

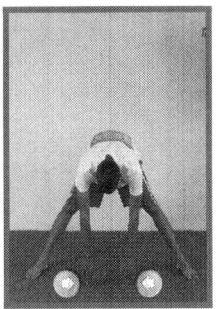

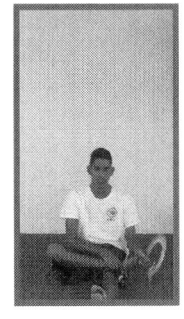

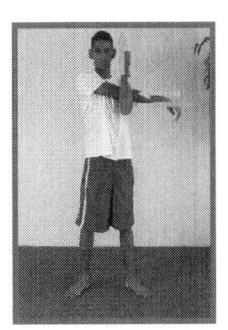

MASTER DENNIS W. BARBEAU
5th Degree Martial Arts Black Belt - Master Instructor

Copyright © 2015 Barbeau Productions LLC

All rights reserved.

ISBN-13: 978-1505287189

ISBN-10: 1505287189

DEDICATION

I would first like to dedicate this book to my mother, Bertha E. Barbeau and father, William J. Barbeau for being my first teachers who instilled in me the martial arts tenets of courtesy, integrity, perseverance, self-control and indomitable spirit. They instilled in me that peace and harmony, which happen to also be the primary goals of a martial artist, were also the principal guides in life which I have always strived to live.

I would also like to dedicate this book to my wife, Sandy, for her patient and loving support, and who has endured daily questions and discussions during the development and construction of this book, and my two wonderful sons, Sean and Ryan, who trained in the martial arts with me, and who have inspired and assisted me in this endeavor with their consistent and patient assistance, consultation, love and support.

Finally, I would like to dedicate this book to my remarkable daughters-in-law, Carlene and Daphna, and my grandchildren, Zachary, Ellie and my new expected grandson yet to be born April 2015, all of whom always give me much love, motivation, support, and many laughs to brighten my days.

CONTENTS

	Dedication	3
	Acknowledgments	5
1	Forward by *Daniel O'Donnell PT, Cert. MDT*	6
2	Introduction	8
3	About This Book	10
4	Stretching & Fitness Routines for Everyone: An Easy Guide To Health	12
5	Standing Stretches	13
6	Preparation & Helpful Stretching Tips	13
7	Trunk (Waist) & Neck Stretches	15
8	Side Muscle Stretches (Side Bends)	19
9	Shoulder Stretches (Arm Circles)	20
10	Rotator Cuff Stretches - Arm Extenders	26
11	Oblique Muscle, Back & Toe Touching Stretches	30
12	Standing leg Stretches	33
13	"Down & Back" Stretches	40
14	Floor (Sitting) Leg Stretches	42
15	Breathing Tips & Stretching - Trunk (Sitting) Open Leg/Back	47
16	Partner (Sitting) Stretches	65
17	Strength Exercises - Push-ups, Sit-ups	68
18	Ending Exercises, Charts & Final Words	79
19	About The Author	88

ACKNOWLEDGMENTS

I would like to acknowledge the following people who assisted in some substantial way in the creation of this project. They are, in no particular order, Sandy Barbeau, Sean Barbeau, Ryan Barbeau, Carlene Barbeau, Daphna Barbeau, Zachary Barbeau, Ellie Barbeau, new baby Barbeau (April 2015), Jaaved K. Khan, Matthew A. Adan, Daniel O'Donnell and Rishika Khan. Special congratulations and appreciation to Jaaved K. Khan and Matthew A. Adan for their total dedication, dependability, and generous offering of their time, effort and friendship in the making and production of this book,

Stretching & Fitness Routines For Everyone:
An Easy Guide To Health

FOREWORD
BY DANIEL O'DONNELL, PT, CERT. MDT

As the reader well knows, the number of books written about some type of exercise is exhaustive. While all authors are presumed to be well intending, many books are written without much science to substantiate the information conveyed in their book. This is the very reason there are so many books written about the same type of exercise; everybody is willing to publish their opinion.

It is therefore satisfying to know there are some authors that not only apply an evidenced-based approach to movement strategies but also bring vast personal experience on which movement prescriptions are based. Master Dennis Barbeau is one of these authors.

The techniques with which Master Barbeau instructs his students are proven effective and most importantly safe movement patterns. They provide all students, including martial arts practitioners, with the necessary flexibility for them to move well and in universally functional progressions.

It is unanimously agreed that the most trying time for an athlete is not learning a skill or the effort of developing powerful movement. Rather, it is that time period of recovery from an injury. In this book, Master Barbeau attends expertly to technique and uses sound, safe progressions when describing the specific movements. This attention to the details of movement greatly reduces risk of injury and therefore the distress of recovery time.

Knowing Master Dennis Barbeau personally and professionally for many years allows me to confidently endorse the content of this, his most recent book. It is refreshing that a man as principled and sincere as Master Barbeau offers to prepare an athlete for competition in a format that brings personal consideration for the athlete's well-being.

It is my enthusiastic pleasure to recommend the reader apply these tactics and precautions as they are described. They are biochemically correct and anatomically accurate. These movements will serve the athlete throughout their competitive career as well as recreational or fitness endeavors. Following through with his fundamentally safe and effective movement instruction ensures success in training of any athlete.

Well done, Dennis. Best of luck to your students.

Daniel O'Donnell, PT, Cert. MDT
Physical Therapist
Certified in Mechanical Diagnosis and Therapy

INTRODUCTION

As a teacher of martial arts for over twenty years, I have always had a dream to share my passion and knowledge of sports and particularly the martial arts. Anyone may benefit from doing these stretching exercises in preparing for their own sports activity. The stretching exercises shown in this book are used and have been used for years personally by me and by my martial arts students. However, they are so effective, I wanted to share them with you and everyone who reads this book and who wants to be more flexible and move more easily throughout their daily activities, whether normal or extreme.

You do not have to be a martial artist to enjoy the benefits of the stretching exercises in this book. Beginners and veterans can benefit by following the clear directions and photographs of these stretching exercises before beginning any activity requiring some muscle preparation.

I am happy now to provide an easy and inexpensive way for interested kids and adults to learn all about preparing the body for doing sports including the martial arts. Furthermore, the reader will discover here an easy-to-read guidebook which shows over 180 photographs with step-by-step instructions on proper stretching and safe preparation of the body to minimize injury and maximize performance in doing most sports.

This book focuses specifically on the proper stretching of the muscles, tendons and ligaments of the body used in sports. Each page describes and shows the proper form and the accurate position of the stretching body part, and guiding arrows show the direction and correct range of motion for the stretches. Stretching exercises will begin in the order used by most instructors and professional coaches, depending on the sports activity involved. The reader may decide to omit or to emphasize certain exercises depending on the sports activity being enjoyed.

I am indebted to Mr. Daniel O'Donnell who lent his expertise in the review of my book to assure readers receive the most updated exercise and fitness information backed by scientific research and experience. Thank you, Dan, once again for your able professional assistance.

<u>NOTE</u>: The reader assumes all the responsibility and all risks in using and following the instructions in this book, and through its purchase, hereby releases the author and all his associates of any liability whatsoever for reckless or incorrect application of its contents.

As always, we wish you safe and happy training and much satisfaction as you gain the knowledge, joy, happiness and good health which comes from proper stretching and preparing to do sports or other dynamic or energetic activities.

Master Dennis W. Barbeau
5th degree black belt, Tae Kwon Do
Certified: Kukkiwon-World Tae Kwon Do Federation, Seoul, S. Korea
2nd degree black belt, Hapkido
Certified: Hapkido International, San Diego, CA
Website: karatekidsconnection.com

ABOUT THIS BOOK
Welcome to
Stretching & Fitness Routines For Everyone - An Easy Guide To Health

This book introduces the new athlete to the basic stretches and flexibility exercises practiced by athletes of most all sports. Anyone of any age can learn and benefit from reading this book. This book is not intended to be or should be understood to give medical advice of any kind. The author is not a medical doctor or medical health professional. The author's intention is only to impart his many years of personal experience in teaching these stretches and techniques, and using his knowledge as both a practitioner and instructor of the martial arts. As with any new activity, interested students should check with their doctors before beginning any new exercise program or if the exercise causes any pain or discomfort. It is also recommended that students begin these stretches slowly and easily. Beginning students are both cautioned and encouraged to not force any stretch, and let the body gradually adapt to the stretch over time as the stretching becomes easier and some results are experienced. These stretches should not cause any significant pain while doing. Of course, students are wise to use this book while seeking out a qualified instructor for the most applicable information to their activity goals, and to reduce the potential for accidental injuries.

This training book is intended as a guide to help you understand how to prepare your body for most sports. These techniques have been and can be successfully applied specifically for anyone training in the martial arts. Some preparation exercises may apply more to martial arts training but, as noted in the book's introduction, they are confidently and successfully used for other sports body preparation as well. The stretching exercises shown here are used by most all professional sports athletes to prepare their bodies for moderate to strenuous activity and to keep their bodies safe from injury. There are many different kinds of stretches. Not all stretches available are shown in this training book because of space. These stretches are also used successfully by anyone, including this author, as preparation to weight lifting and training to target, loosen and prepare those body parts needed for particular lifts. Readers interested in dieting, weight loss programs, running, jogging, bicycling, and many other activities can benefit by doing these stretches both before and after training.

Unlike our earlier book, **Karate Kids Connection-Tae Kwon Do Style**, this training book on stretching provides a complete stretching exercise program. Anyone, including current athletes and prospective or veteran martial arts students, can benefit from this book. Although, martial arts students will discover this book specifically outlines most all the stretches and preparation exercises used before martial arts training classes and can be used both before training classes or to review at home those helpful stretches learned in class, the book also helps to get the body ready for the variety of bodily movements used specifically in martial arts activities. However, as mentioned, everyone can use, practice and benefit from all these stretching, flexibility and strength preparation exercises.

It is important to note that there is more than one way to do stretching exercises when preparing for a taxing activity. Proper preparation will depend on the activity, sport, and even the instructor. As noted, the stretching exercises we show here are not exhaustive. There are many kinds of stretching exercises which can be used. We show the exercises here which are typically used by most sports enthusiasts and specifically interested in preparing the body for more active training and activity. Again, these same exercises can be used by anyone preparing for any strenuous activity.

It is generally noted that before any extreme activity, especially those movements requiring fast, sudden bursts of energy or what are normally referred to as ballistic movements, stretching alone is not sufficient to prepare those muscle groups. More thorough range-of-motion movements should be done prior to these more demanding, sudden movements.

It is important to note here that for those students preparing for martial arts activities, such as full contact sparring or fighting, or other activities intended to exert power or force upon an intended target, the stretching exercises shown in this book should first be followed by range-of-motion exercises sometimes known in martial arts classes as drills. **Drills are routines where certain body parts (i.e., arms, legs, etc.) are used in repetitive motions, forcing repeated actions of certain muscle groups, specific muscles, tendons and ligaments in a non-ballistic movement pattern. These range-of-motion movements are done more moderately before using those muscles and muscle groups for more intense, full power exertion on a prospective target.**

<u>**IMPORTANT NOTE**</u>: **Be patient with yourself when doing all stretches. In time, with consistent training and patience, you will gain increased flexibility and without undue pain while avoiding unnecessary injury. Go slow, be patient, and experience the benefits.**

STRETCHING & FITNESS ROUTINES FOR EVERYONE

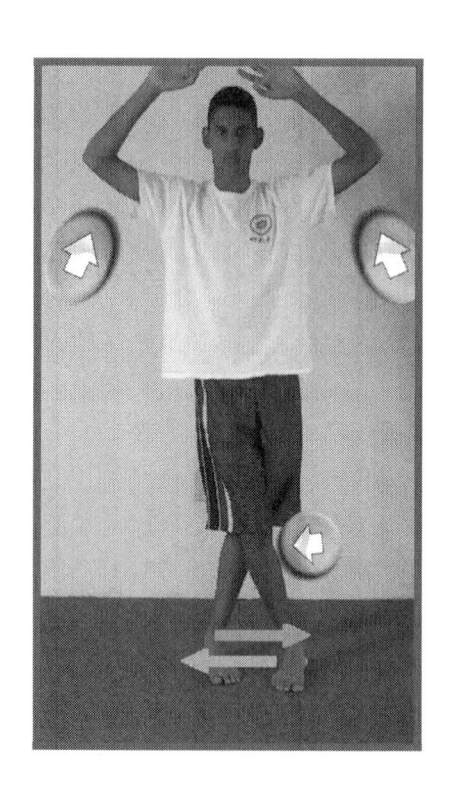

AN EASY GUIDE TO HEALTH

STANDING STRETCHES

PREPARATION

Although I will be teaching the preparatory stretches in the typical order used in many martial arts classes, the student will notice that some stretches are not necessarily done in this order. Generally, stretching exercises usually begin with first stretching the larger muscle groups. Therefore, we are going to begin our exercises with the larger body movements.

Before beginning the stretching activities, it is recommended to always begin with a light run or jogging exercise. Lightly jogging before stretching warms up the muscles, begins the stretching of the ligaments and tendons in the arms and legs, and encourages blood circulation throughout the body in preparation for more strenuous movements. Generally, it is good preparation to jog or lightly run for about 3-5 minutes before beginning the stretching exercises. In bad weather or where space is minimal, simple jumping jacks can be substituted for jogging. I will explain more later on in the book about jumping jacks, and how to create several challenges for yourself with this exercise.

After the initial jogging or run, you can start the more specific stretching exercises. Most stretches are in groups of four to six movements, and are done generally in "forward" and "reverse" directions to move the target muscle or muscle group in both directions through the total "range of movement." It is important to make deliberate motions in as big of circles as you can. This is called moving within the range of motion, which is as far as you should safely move your arms, legs, neck or other joints so that the muscles are stretched and moved safely without injury.

HELPFUL TIPS ABOUT STRETCHING & BREATHING

For exercises requiring bending, try to first inhale before you bend, then exhale when bending into the stretch. When you transition to the next stretch, again inhale when leaving the earlier stretch, and exhale when reaching for the next stretch. For brevity, I will not repeat this tip with each exercise description, but try to remember to follow it since it applies to all stretching exercises. When you stretch it helps to count by saying 1001 (one thousand and one, etc.), 1002, 1003, 1004, 1005, etc. When you say 1001, it is like holding the stretch for a full second of time. Depending on the body part being stretched, you can hold a stretch for 4-10 seconds for a good stretch, which you should repeat three or four times. NOTE: the current research suggests one 30-second sustained muscle stretch is optimum.

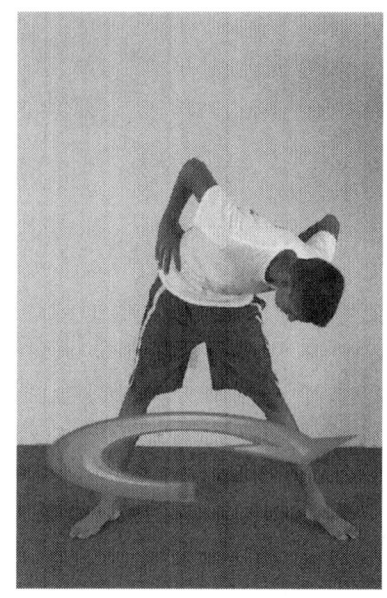

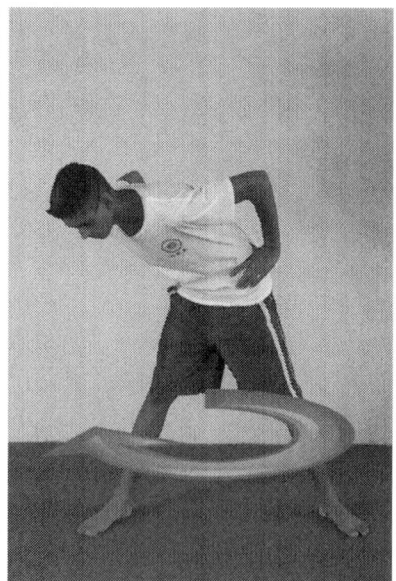

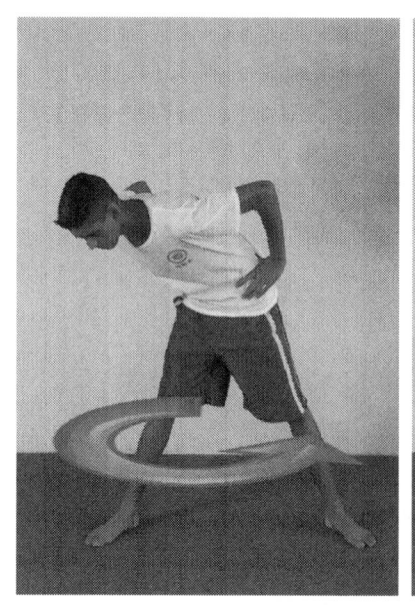

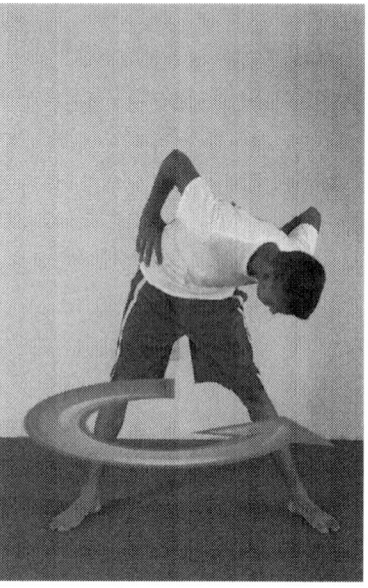

Trunk (Waist) Stretches

TRUNK (WAIST) STRETCHES

After kicking/shaking our legs and feet lightly for a few seconds and simultaneously lightly shaking our arms and hands, we first begin with the large trunk exercise. The trunk is your waist which supports the top of your body including your abdomen, chest, shoulders, arms, back, neck and head. We refer to the stretching of these body parts primarily as trunk exercises. We first make large circular movements at the waist by moving the entire top of the body in large circles. (See previous page). Begin by placing your hands on your hips and moving the top of your body in both directions. Placing your hands on your hips gives support and stability to the circular movement. You can see in the pictures that the student is moving his body, making large circles with his upper body as it turns on the hips. Repeat this trunk stretch for four complete circle movements in each direction.

NECK STRETCHES

Once this trunk exercise is complete, continue the circular movements with your neck. The average adult head weighs about 10-11 pounds. The neck's job is to support the head. However, it is made of many relatively small bones and is quite easily injured. Careful preparation of the neck muscles is important for conditioning and strengthening of the neck to minimize potential injury. You will want to keep this in mind when exercising and stretching the neck muscles. These stretches are shown in detail on the next three pages. Remember to avoid forcing extension of the neck in any direction.

Keep your hands on your waist at your sides. Again, you will want to complete about four circular movements in each direction, as shown in the pictures below. It is helpful to transition to this neck stretch by moving the neck in the circular direction as you were moving the final trunk stretching movement. So if you were moving your upper body in a clockwise direction for the final movement, you would continue the first circular neck movement in the same direction as you transition to the neck muscle stretch.

When the circular neck stretches are completed, keeping your hands on your waist at your sides, gently lower your chin to your chest and hold for 5-10 seconds. Then gently raise your head back, lifting your chin.

Neck Circle Stretches

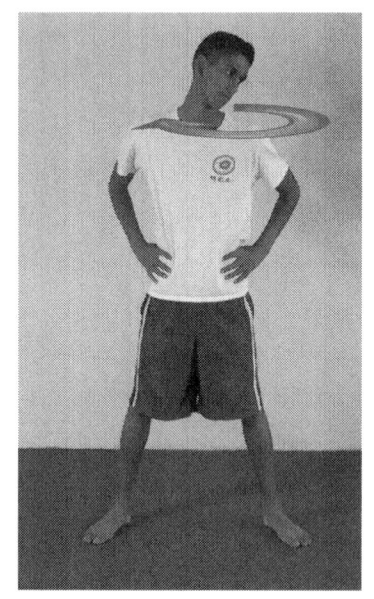

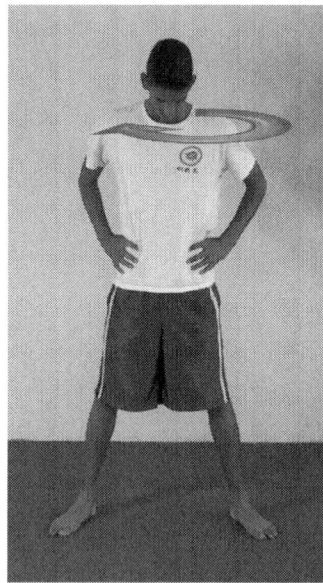

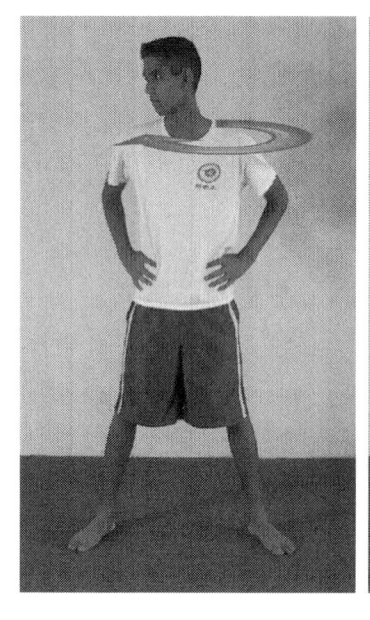

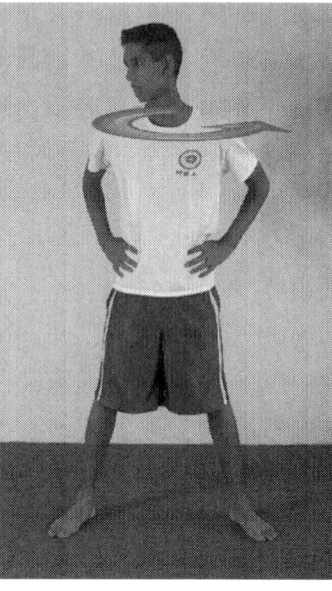

Neck Forward/Back Tilting Stretches

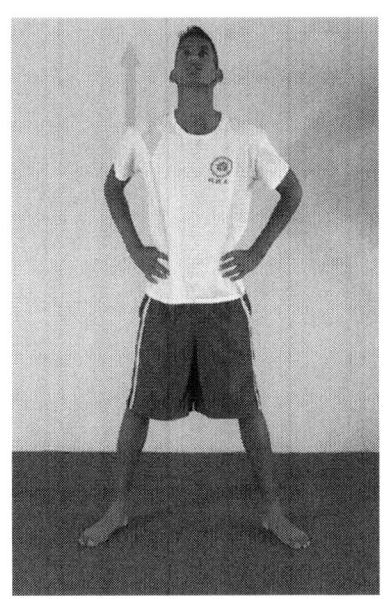

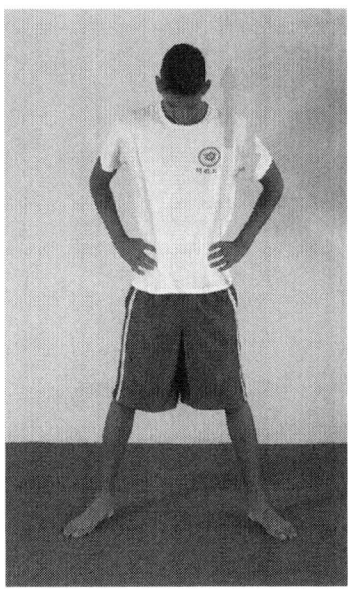

Neck Side-to-Side Tilting Stretches

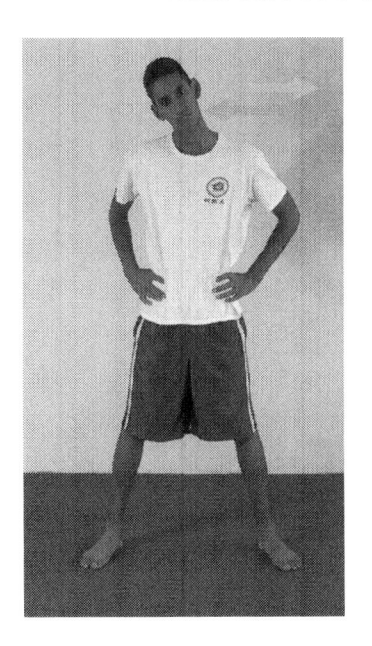

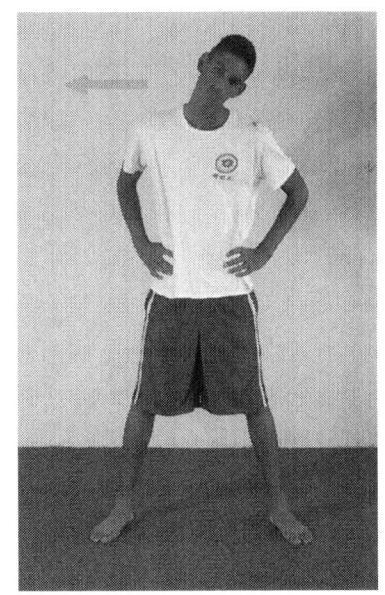

Neck Turning Stretches

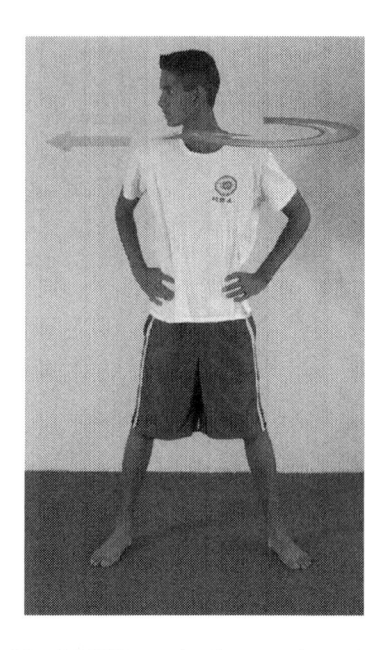

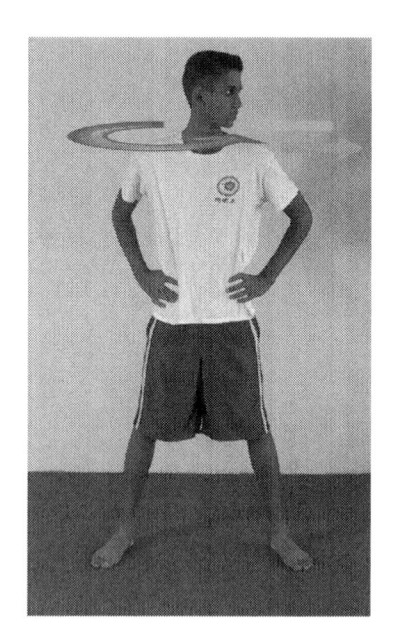

Do NOT push the neck or head forcefully with this stretch. This will help avoid hyper-extension of the neck and excessive pressure on the back of the neck which could cause injury. Carefully repeat this forward and back exercise two or three times.

Once this stretch is completed, keeping your hands on your waist return your head to the normal, straight forward position and turn your head looking to one side, and hold for a few seconds. Switch the stretch and look to the opposite side and hold. Repeat this exercise two or three times.

Once this stretch is completed, tilt your head to the side and hold again for a few seconds, and again switch the tilt direction to the opposite side and hold. Repeat this side to side stretch two or three times.

The final neck stretch is the "chin to chest to shoulder" stretch. For this stretch lower your chin to your chest while continuing an upward motion toward the shoulder, and back again to the chest and opposite shoulder. Repeat this stretch two or three times, ending with one complete circular head rotation followed by the opposite full 360 degree rotation. Again, as mentioned earlier, you will want to be careful not to push the head backward too forcefully, again to avoid injury to the neck.

SIDE MUSCLE STRETCHES (SIDE BENDS)

After stretching your trunk and your neck, your next upper body stretch requires you place your hands on your hips with feet about shoulder-width apart. Begin this stretch by bending to one side, If you bend to your right side, take your left arm and reach directly over your head as if to touch your right ear as you bend to the right. Hold for 3-4 seconds, then switch. Bend to your left side, taking your right hand and reach over your head for your left ear, and hold for 3-4 seconds. Repeat this sequence three of four times, and return to center (standing upright position.) Never bounce with your stretch. Always pull steadily and relax your muscles when pulling gently. This provides for a steady, static stretch rather than a ballistic, or bouncing, movement for a much better stretch.

Side Bend Stretches

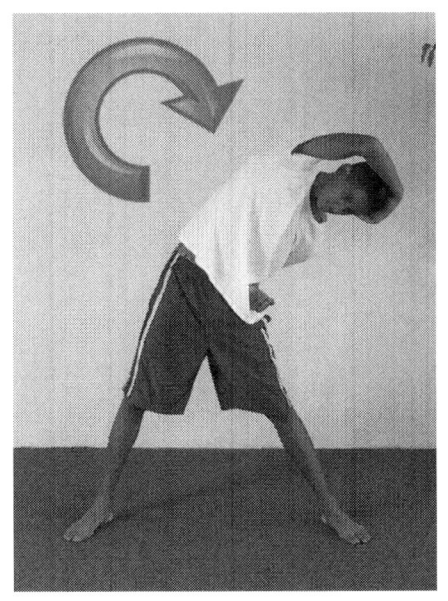

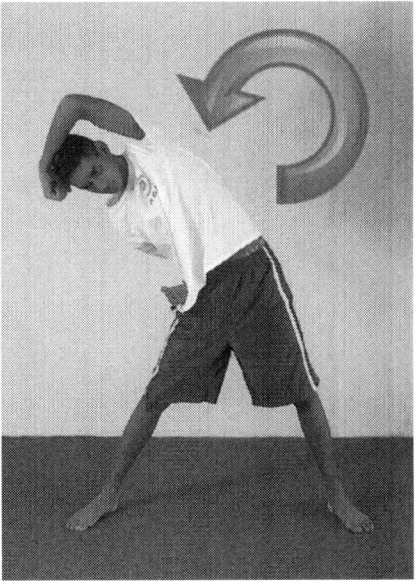

SHOULDER STRETCHES (ARM CIRCLES)

After stretching your trunk, neck and sides, you will proceed to the next upper but smaller muscle groups of the shoulders and arms. For the shoulder stretches, extend your arms in front of your body and make slow, as large as possible circular movements, moving both arms in a vertical direction and in forward circles, in an upward and downward circular direction. Then reverse the direction, swinging your arms in a similar backward motion.

Begin with your arms/palms extended as far as possible straight out in front of you, palms facing upward. As you lift your arms upward, palms up, breathe in through your nose and begin a circular movement overhead. As you reach the top of the circular stretch and proceed backward (or sideward,) turn palms downward and begin to exhale through your mouth as your arms extend outward and downward to your sides to begin another rotation. Do this stretch two or three times.

Arm Circle Stretches

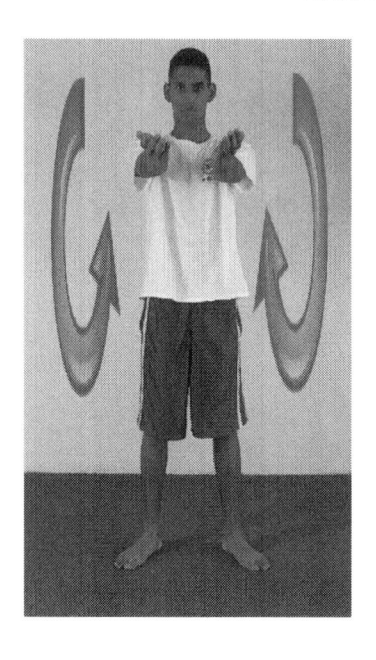

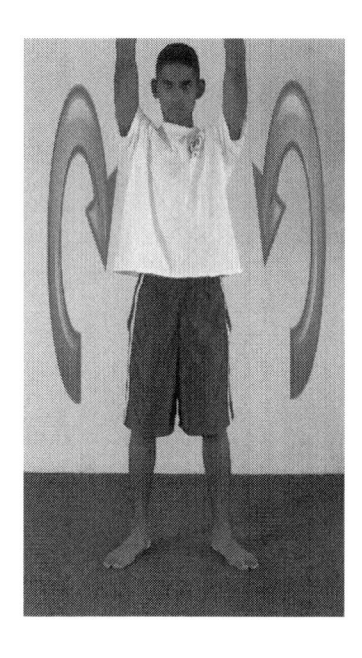

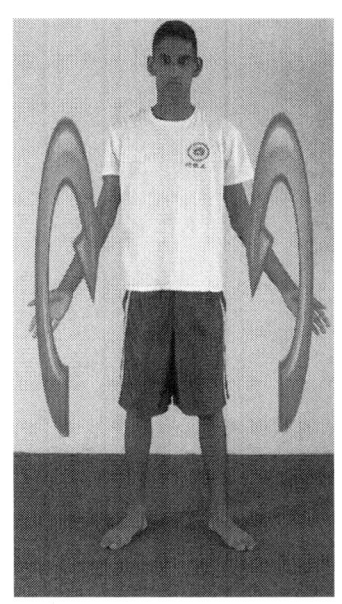

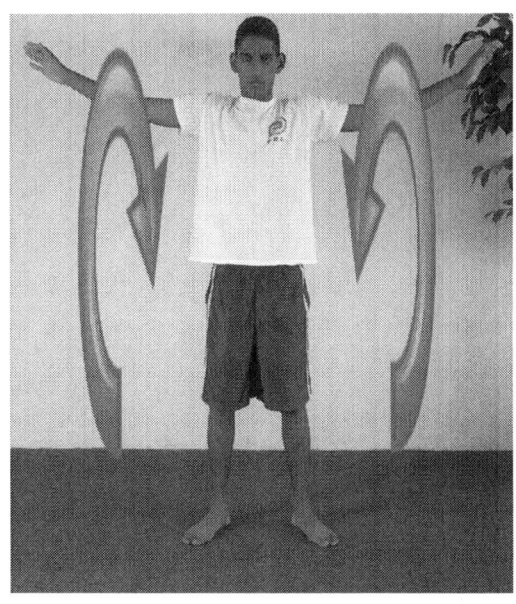

Arm Circle Stretches - reverse motion

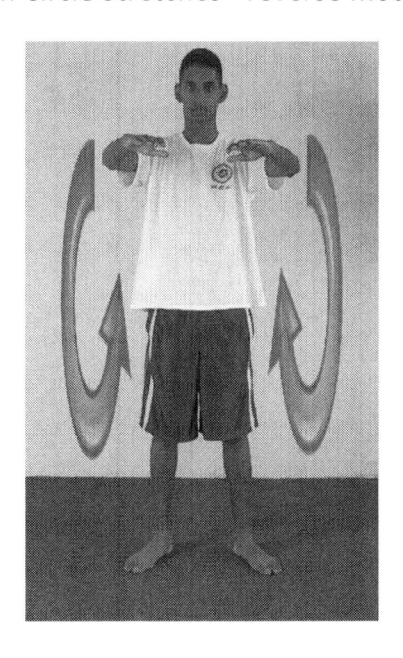

Now reverse the movement. This time begin with your arms at your sides. Lift your arms from your sides, palms facing upward and inhale again through the nose. As you bring them toward the front of your body, turn palms downward and push outward, exhaling through your mouth, to get as good a stretch as possible. Repeat these circular forward and backward stretches three of four times in each direction. Because your shoulder blades prevent your arms from fully extending behind you, swing your arms without force in both directions to get the full benefit of the shoulder stretch. These shoulder stretches are very important. They not only stretch the shoulder muscles but also put the rotator cuffs through maximum range of motion to prepare and protect the delicate ligaments and tendons in these shoulder joints. For additional benefit, you can swing your arms in opposite directions simultaneously. Swimmers often use this type of shoulder stretch. Allow these stretches to be free and easy. Do not force these circular movements. Relax your shoulders and arms when stretching.

Arm/Chest/Back Across Stretches

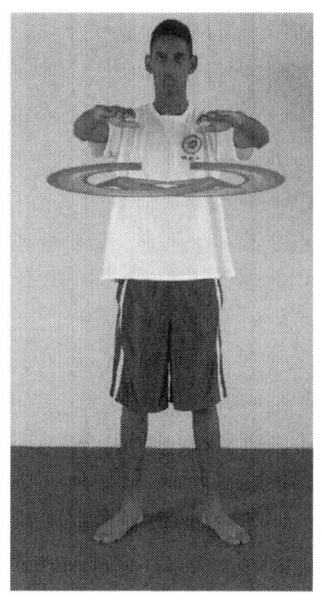

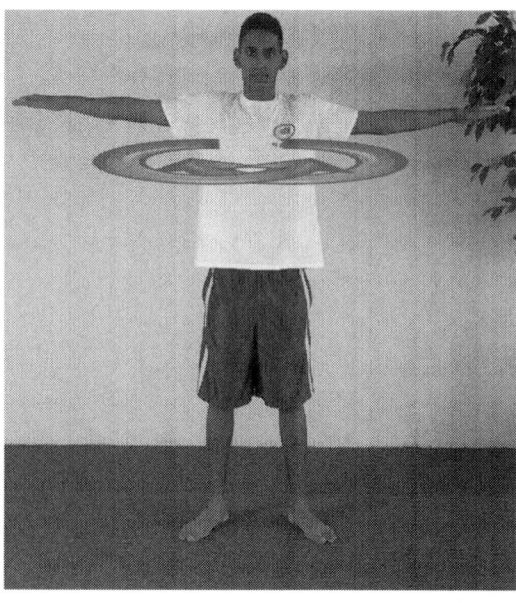

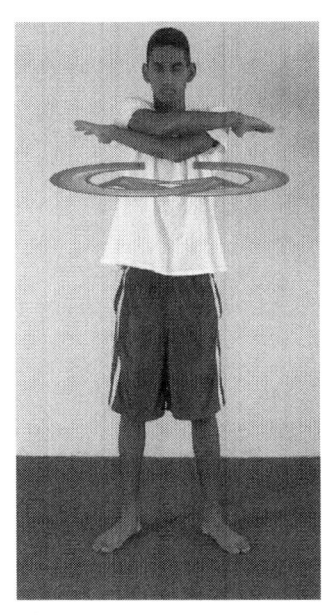

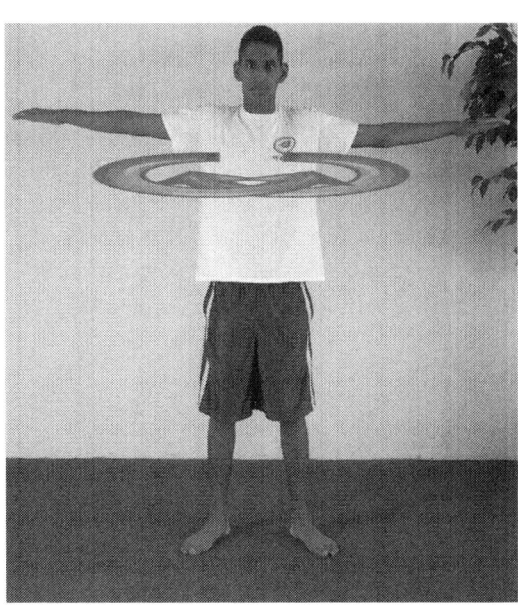

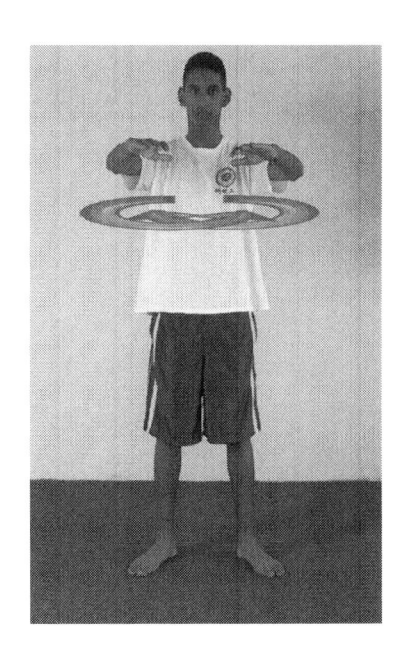

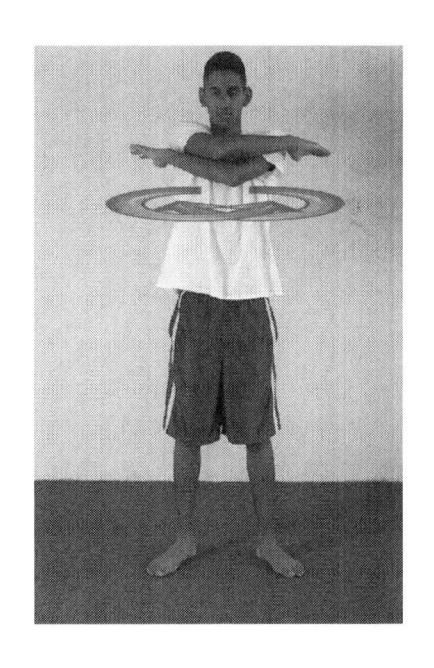

After vertically stretching your shoulders, continue the circular motion on a horizontal plane directly in front of your chest. Swing each arm directly sideways and out to its fullest extension, then while keeping them extended swing your arms to the opposite side, crossing the elbows in front of your chest (see previous page). When extending your arms to the sides, push your arms out as far as possible and swing them outward enough to feel the stretch in your pectoral (chest) muscles, and hold for the stretch. Then bring your arms back and cross them in front of your chest, reaching for the opposite side or even shoulder blade if you can reach that far. You will be stretching the large muscles in your back also with this move. You will inhale through the nose on the outward swing, and exhale through your mouth on the cross stretch. Remember to keep your arms parallel to the floor for the maximum benefit on each movement. There is a tendency to drop the arms on each swing in and out which will minimize the benefits of the upper body stretch.

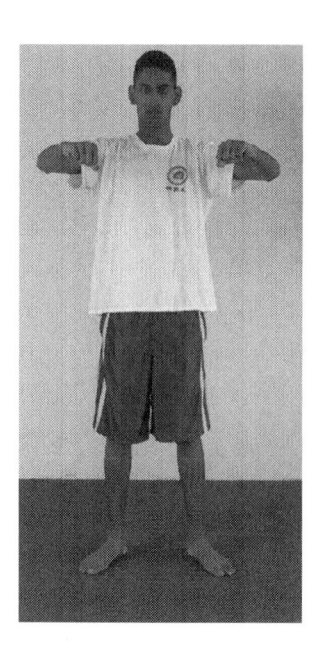

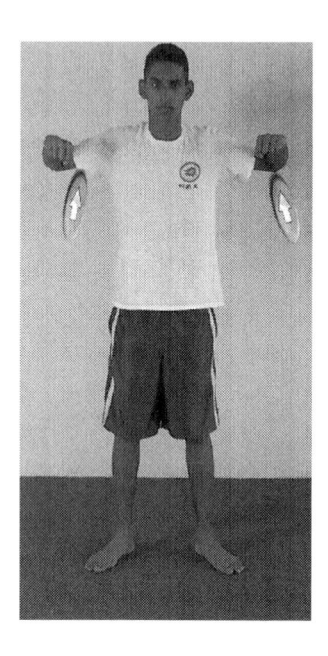

Elbows "up" Stretching

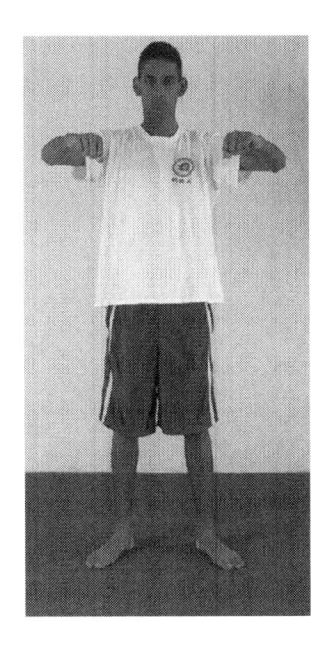

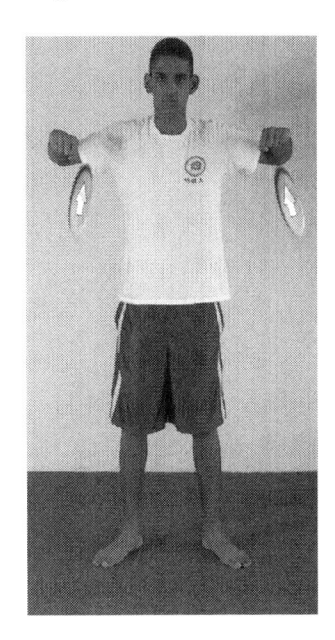

Now keep your arms in the same position but bend your arms so your elbows can be pointed directly backwards and up, arms bent. Simultaneously push both elbows backward to once again stretch the shoulders, bring them forward slightly and repeat a few times. Be sure to leave your arms parallel to the floor when stretching the elbows backward for the best stretch. Then, make a fist and turning your palms upward with arms bent, elbows next to your sides, and push your elbows straight back and upward, as if poking someone in the side, Push both arms backward as far as possible, simultaneously bringing them forward and backward several times. When you complete all these shoulder/arm exercises, you can repeat any or all of these exercises at your discretion in a series of free movements, shaking and moving them to "shake out" any stiffness or discomfort. You can now proceed to the next exercise.

ROTATOR CUFF STRETCHES / ARM EXTENDERS

Once all these shoulder circle exercises are completed, you now will exercise and stretch each arm/rotator cuff separately. Take one arm and raise it over your head, bending the elbow, as if to touch the back of your neck or between your shoulder blades.

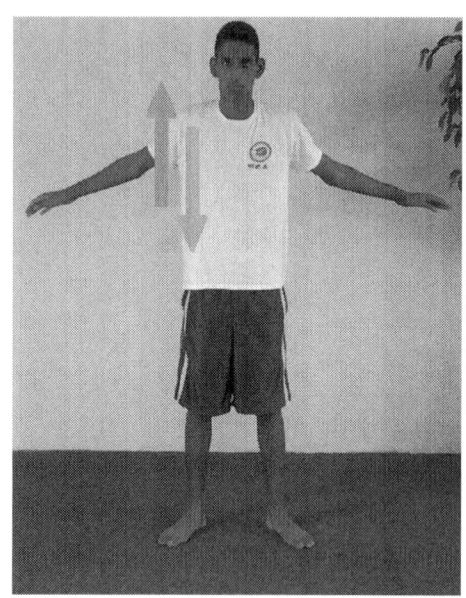

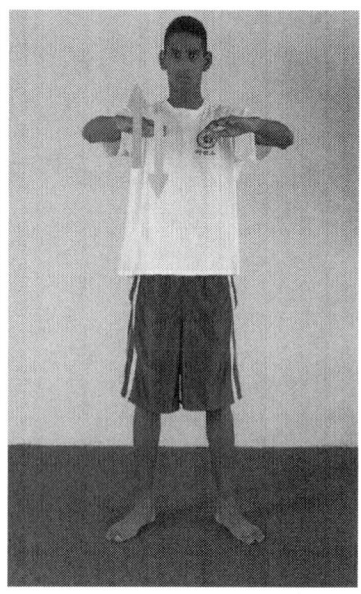

With your elbow now pointing upward and your hand behind your neck, take your other hand and gently pull your raised elbow backward to aid in the stretch. If you can pat your back with the stretching arm, you are doing it correctly. Hold this stretch for about 5-10 seconds. Allow this same arm to drop and forward and swing across your chest to the opposite side. Grab and support this arm, cradling your arm with the other arm in the bend of the elbow and while making a fist, as if to do a bicep squeeze. Again, hold for about 5-10 seconds. Swing the arm downward, and once again allow the arm to return to behind the head position, again pulling slightly backward with the opposite hand. You can repeat this stretch two or three times. Then, switch arms. See the pictures here and the next page.

Arm Back-Elbow-Up, Rotator Cuff Stretch

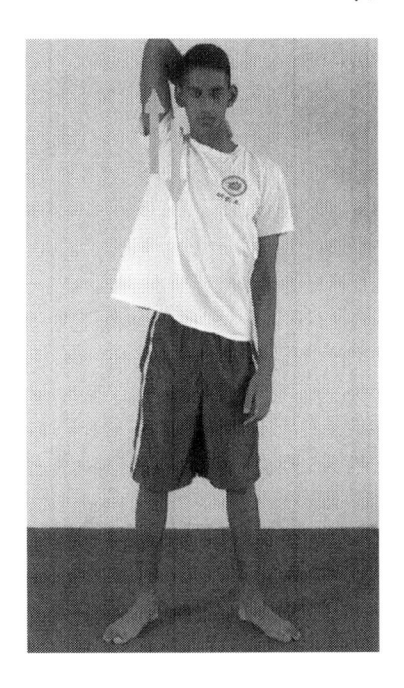

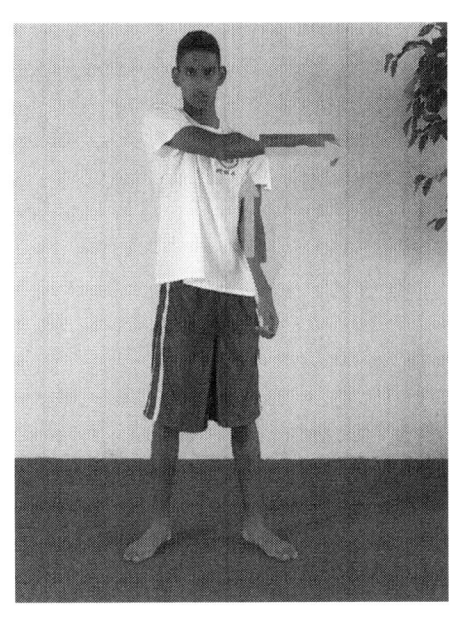

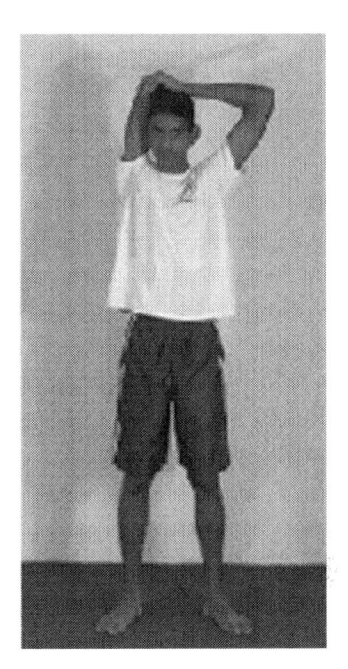

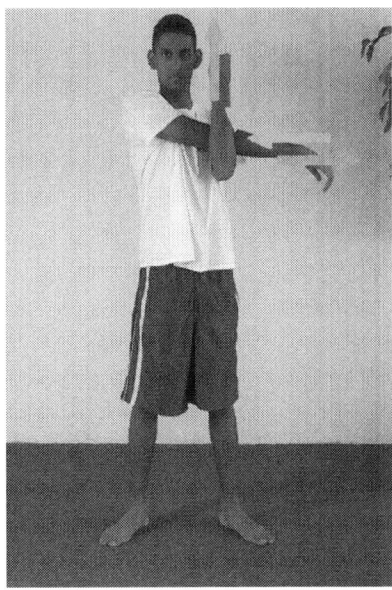

Now swing the opposite arm behind the head, pull and support, and swing across the chest (arm extenders), as you did with the first arm, repeating this stretching combination two or three times. When finished stretching both arms behind your head and across your chest, move both arms freestyle in forward and backward circles to "shake out" the stretch, allowing your muscles to relax. Note: advanced students may want to also extend each arm horizontally behind the back for additional rotator cuff stretching.

Switch Arms - Same Arm Back-Elbow-Up Stretches

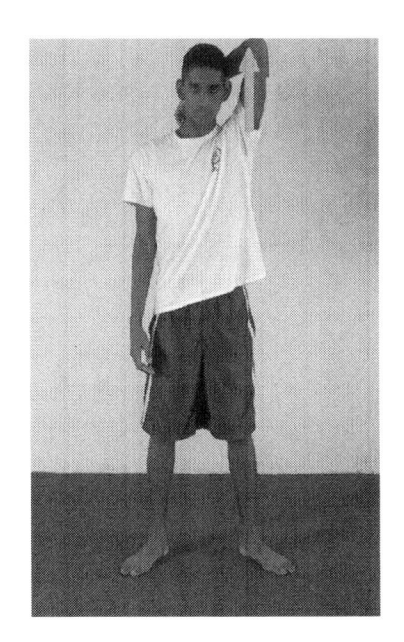

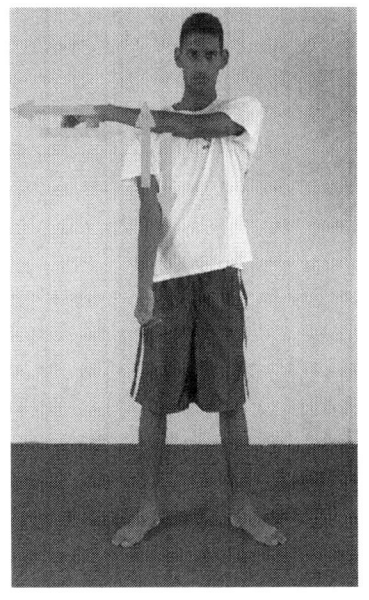

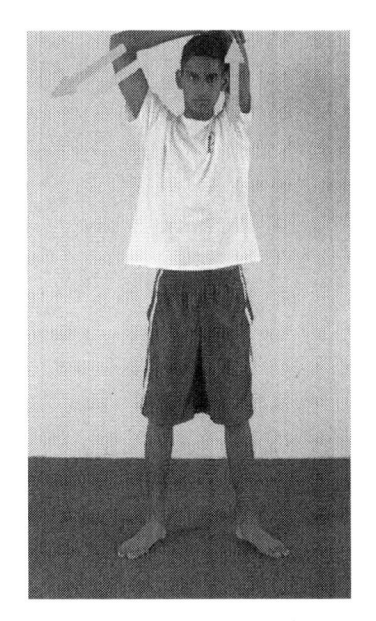

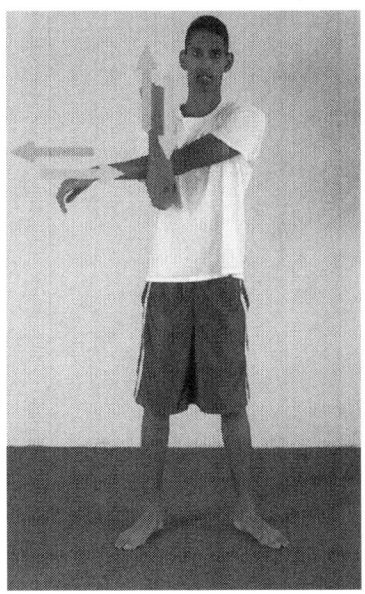

OBLIQUE MUSCLE STRETCHES (SIDE TURNS)

The next exercise if to stretch the oblique or side/back muscles. These are large muscles which extend from the side, around to your back. These muscles are strong muscles and are used in martial arts for torqueing and preparing to execute a martial arts kick, as well as other upper body punches and strikes. To begin this exercise, take your hands and lock them in front of your abdomen. Lock your hand by making a fist and placing the fingers of each hand inside the other hand, as if to "hook" them inside the hands (see picture below). Begin by turning to the side as far back as you can turn, looking behind you. For a good stretch, try to look directly behind you and a little further as you stretch and hold this position for 3-4 seconds, Then switch and turn toward the opposite side, again holding for a few seconds (next page). Repeat this stretch in both directions two or three times, and return to center, facing forward. Shake our your arms and lightly kick out your legs to relax these muscles for the next stretch.

Oblique (Side/Back) Muscle Stretches

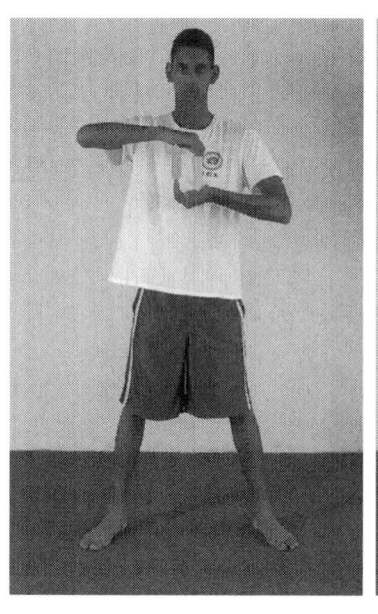

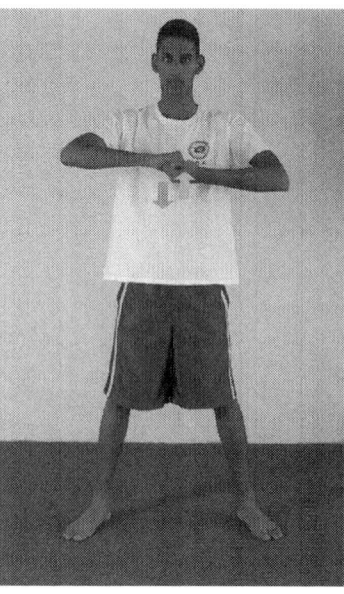

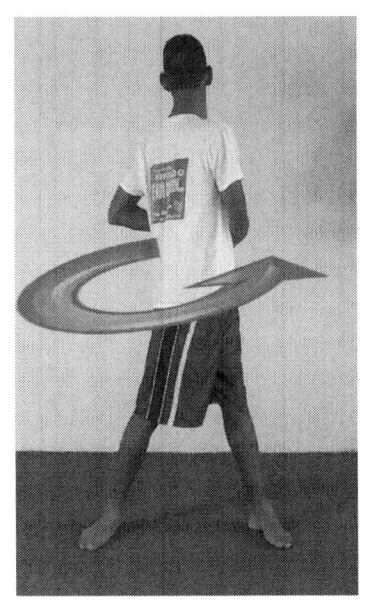

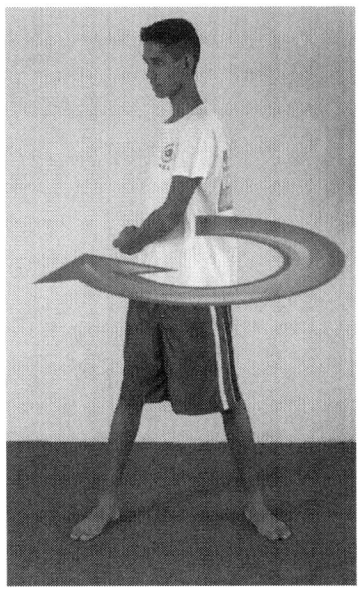

BACK/TOE TOUCH STRETCH

Stand with your ankles together and slightly bend your knees (next page). Lean forward and place your hands on your knees, and hold this stretch for a few seconds. Then reach for your shins and hold for a few seconds. Grab your ankles and hold for a few seconds. With your knees still bent, touch your toes, hold, then the floor with your finger tips and hold. If you feel particularly flexible, try to place your palms on the floor and hold for a few seconds. When finished holding, bring your hands back to your knees, and with knees touching guide your knees in a circle two or three times, then reverse the circular movement in the opposite direction. To assist this circular move, with hands on your knees you can interlock your thumbs for additional support. When you have made two or three circles with your knees in both directions, guide your knees together to make a figure 8. Move in a figure 8 pattern two or three times, then reverse the direction for another two or three patterns. These stretching movements help keep the knee joints flexible and strong. Technically, the knee joints are considered a "simple hinge joint." However, it is important to know that any stretch done outside flexion/extension movements (i.e., twisting to the sides) are not considered safe.

Knee Circle Stretches

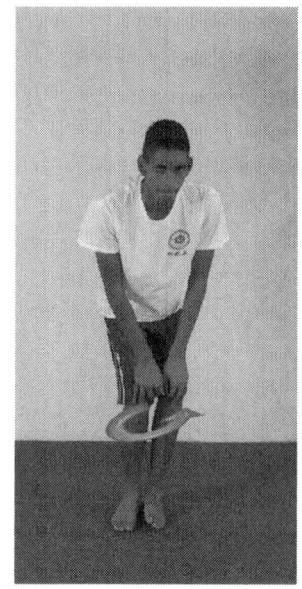

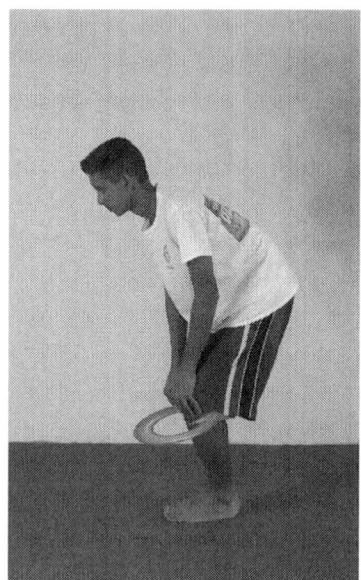

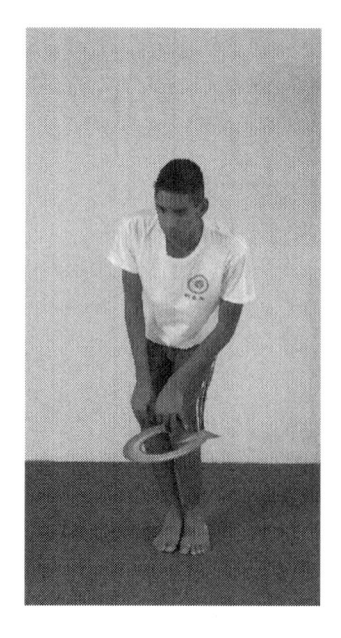

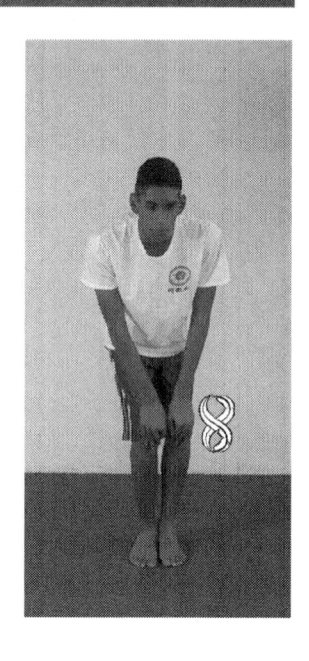

STANDING LEG STRETCHES

At this point in your stretching workout, you have prepared your entire upper body for more active motion. We begin now to stretching of the lower body. You will now continue to stretch your lower back and begin stretching the larger muscles of the legs.

(Note: Since back problems are particularly a problem for some people, you should consult your doctor before beginning any exercises requiring bending or manipulation of the back.)

This next exercise which accomplishes this task begins by spreading each leg out to the side. The distance between stretched legs will vary with each person. However, you will find the distance which is initially comfortable for you, generally about one yard or meter. Begin by stretching your legs out to the sides to a comfortable distance, a little wider than your shoulder width. Hint: the farther you can spread your legs apart, and easier it will be to touch the floor. Bending forward at the waist toward the floor, touch the floor with your fingertips. If you are a beginner or have some difficulty bending forward, you can use a chair or another piece of furniture to help you safely bend forward without hurting yourself, especially your back.

Now reach for your right ankle, placing your hands on or around your right ankle. Hold for 3-4 seconds. Repeat this same stretch on the left side, and this series of right and left stretches two or three times. Next, place your fingertips on your right big toe, and hold for 3-4 seconds. Then switch doing the same stretch on the left side, and hold for a few seconds. Repeat this on both sides two or three times, then place your fingertips on the floor, directly between your feet. For an even better stretch, now spread your legs another inch or two apart on each side, and repeat the series of right and left leg stretches, and return to the middle position, ending with touching the floor with your fingertips.

Standing Leg Side Stretches - Both Hands Floor/Ankle Touch

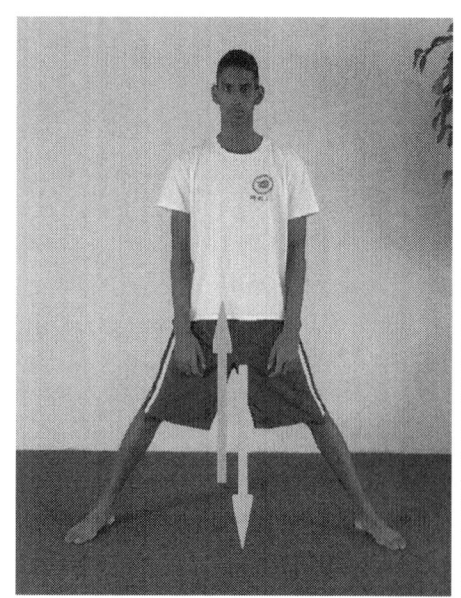

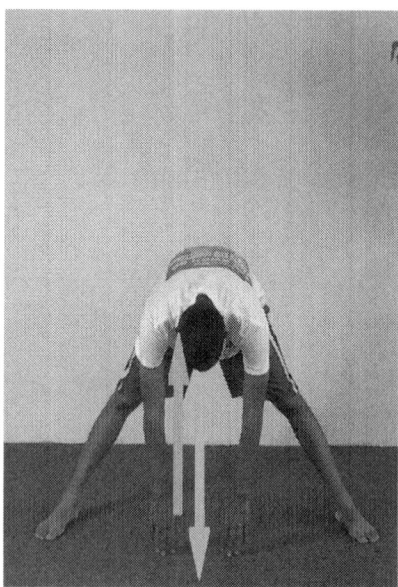

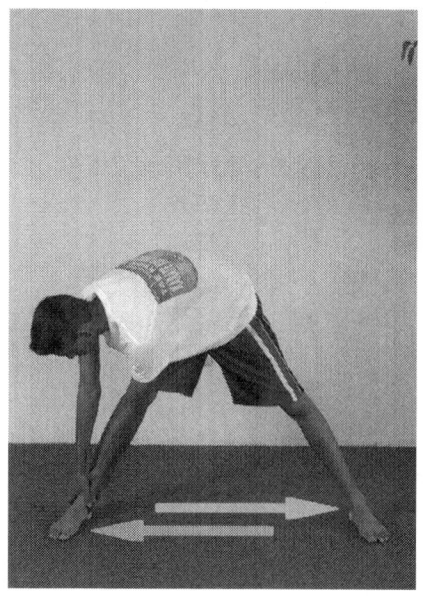

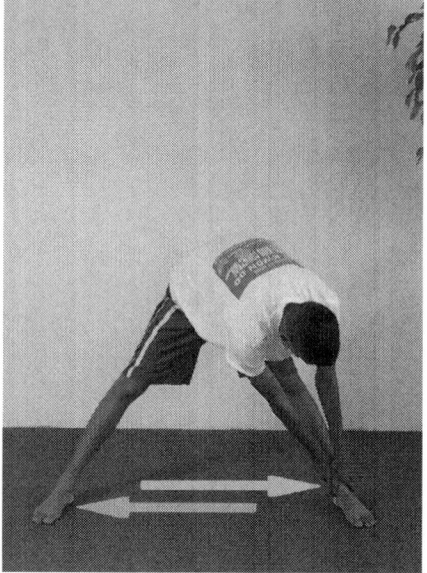

After spreading your legs further apart, repeat the same stretches this time by placing your fingertips on your big toe, and placing your head on your knee each stretch. You can finish this stretch again by placing your fingertips on the floor between your legs, and try putting your "contact" knuckles on the floor. In martial arts the contact knuckles are the large knuckles of the first and middle fingers from the thumb. This stretch adds another couple of inches to your stretch (next page.) You can finish repeating the leg stretches and ending this time with placing your palms on the floor, which again adds an additional challenge to your stretch. You can continue leg stretching by touching the floor with your elbows on the floor if you can, and return to the standing position. If the elbow stretch is too hard for you in the beginning, save that stretch for later when your body feels ready.

Standing Leg Side Stretches
* Both Hands Ankle Touch & Head-on-Knee

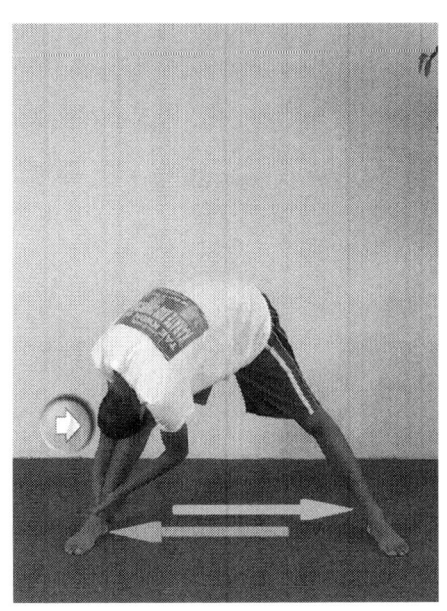

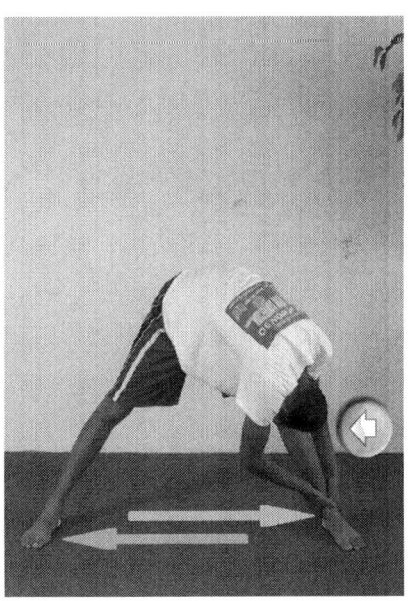

Finger Tip and Palm Floor Touch

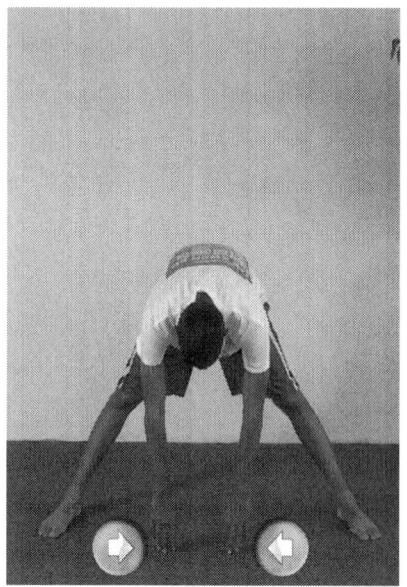

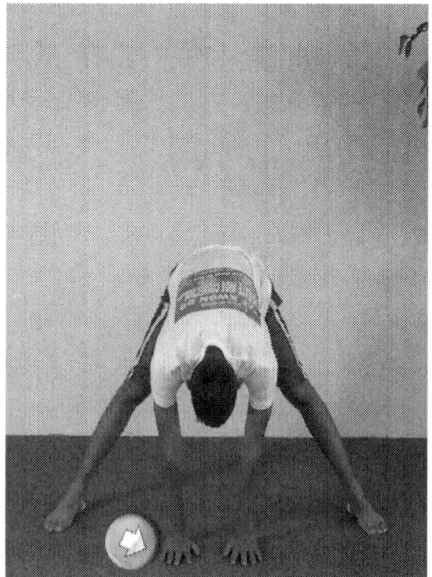

Now, standing with your legs spread apart, grab both your ankles with your hands and lower your head between your legs as far as you can (next page). As you release your grip, slowly bring your feet and ankles together. You can brace yourself by bending the knees and touching the floor if it helps. As you bring your legs together squat down, knees bending, and try to maintain the bottom of your feet flat on the floor while squatting, holding this static position for a few seconds. Using your large leg muscles, now stand and alternately gently kick out our legs to shake the muscles, allowing the muscles to return naturally.

Spread Legs Wider - Repeat Same Leg Stretches with Palms & Knuckle Floor Touches

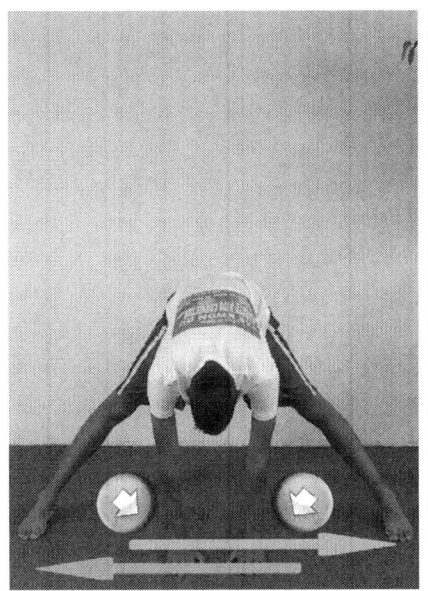

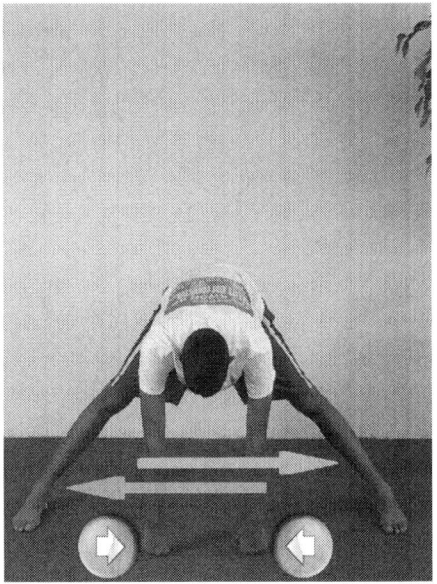

Grab Both Ankles - Lower Head Between Legs

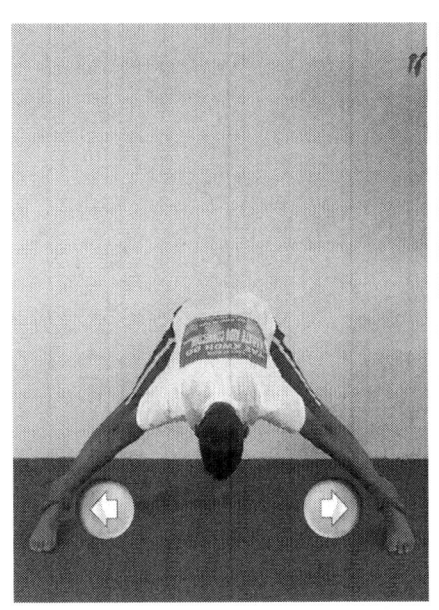

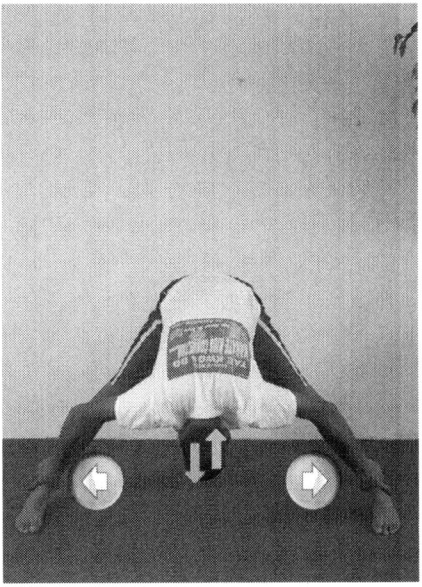

Legs Wide - Repeat Same Leg Stretches Touching Toe, Head on Knee

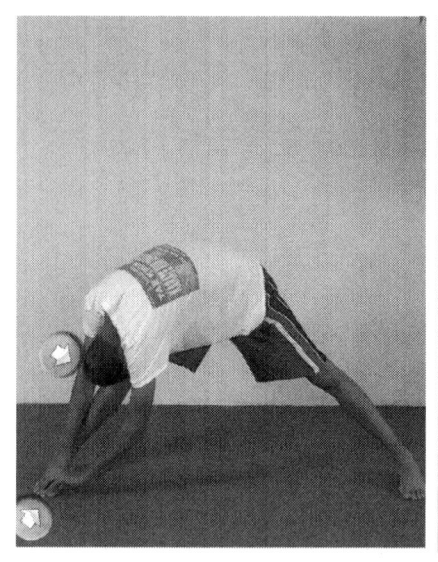

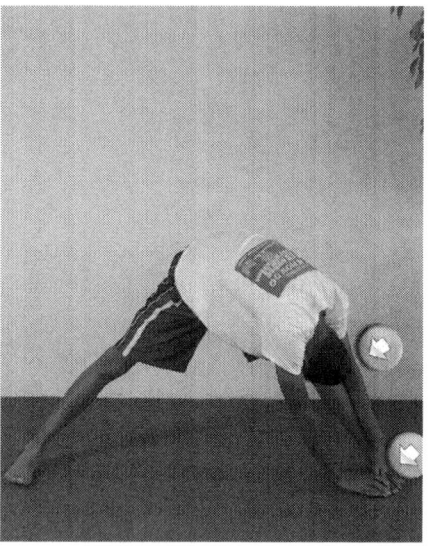

While standing with legs wide apart, without moving your feet, bend your right knee and lower your seat toward and directly above your right ankle as your left leg straightens, resting on the heel, tow up. Then switch sides (see below). Support your weight with your palms on the floor directly in front of you. This same stretch can be done by pointing the toe down. Note: with toe down, care needs to be maintained to keeping the foot straight, and avoid twisting the foot sideways (outside flexion/extension movements). Again, it is important to know that any stretch done outside flexion/extension movements (i.e., twisting to the sides) are not considered safe.

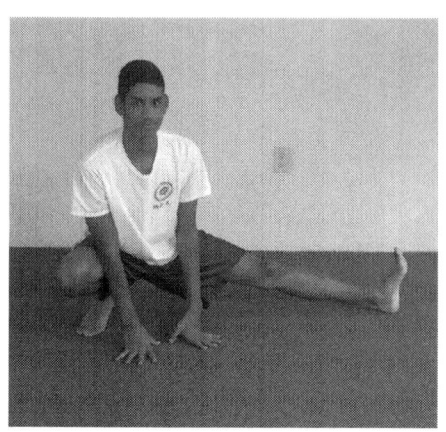

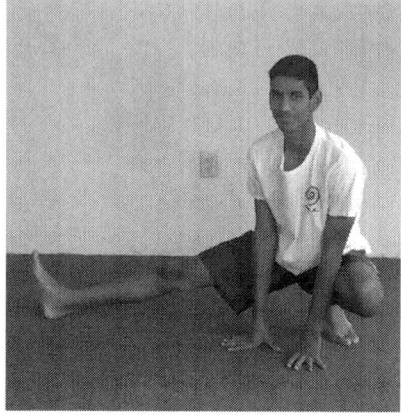

After touching the floor between your legs once again, try to do the side leg stretch. With legs apart, twist your hips to the right and again to the left, with the front leg resting the right heel and the back foot resting on the ball of the foot (directly below the toes), supporting your weight with both hands, one hand in front and one hand in back of your body, as shown below. Be careful not to force the stretch. To widen the stretch even further, wiggle the back foot farther backwards. For the best stretch, remember to keep your knee off the floor.

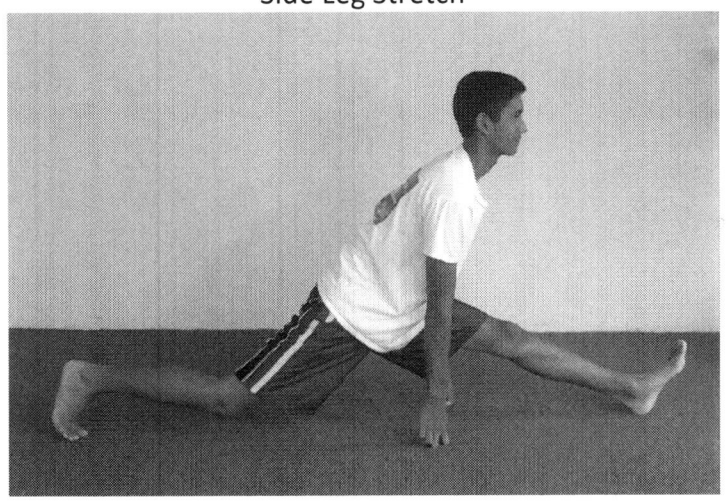

Side Leg Stretch

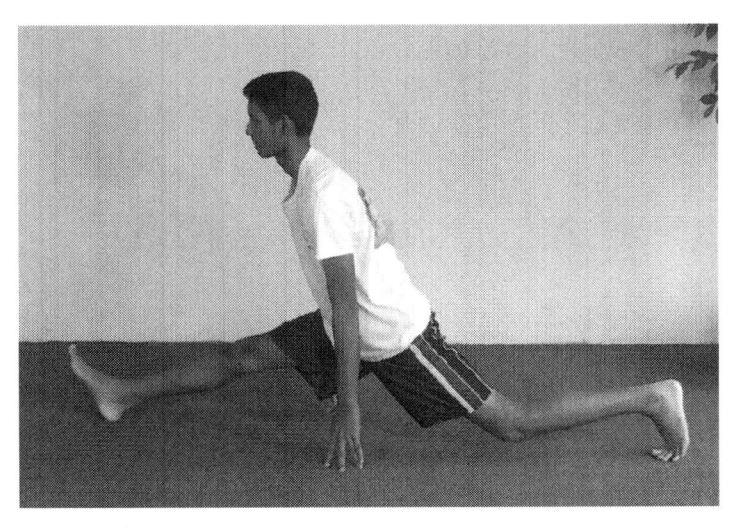

DOWN & BACK STRETCHES

You have stretched out your upper body including your back, arms and waist, and lower body initial leg stretches. You are now ready to begin more active movement stretching. Your next exercise begins with feet spread slightly wider than shoulder width, facing forward. Bend forward and with both hands touch the floor with your fingertips. In the same mild downward effort, continue reaching between your legs and touch the floor as far back as you can reach, then return to an upright position, continuing to lean backward to stretch your back (next page). Repeat this "down and back" stretch two times, with the third and fourth stretch, try to touch your palms to the floor. When completing this exercise, shake out both arms, hands, legs and feet, again to restore and relax them after the stretch.

"Down & Back" Back Bend Stretches

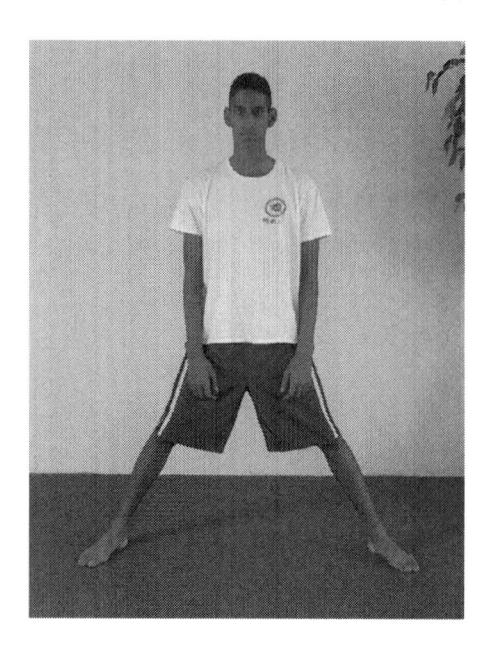

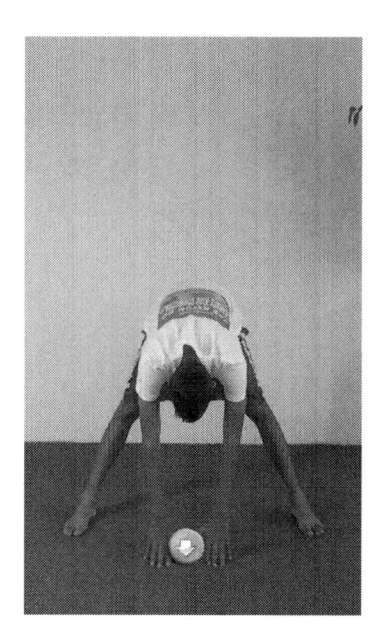

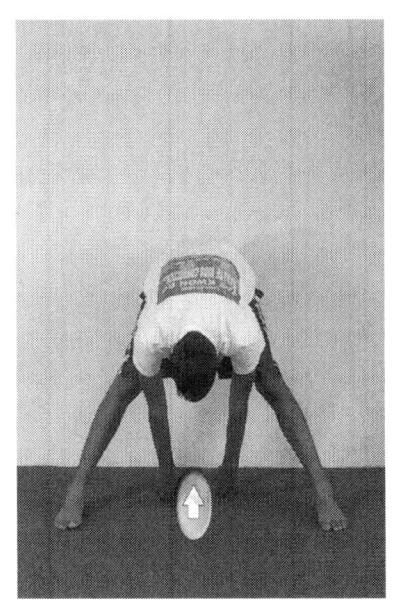

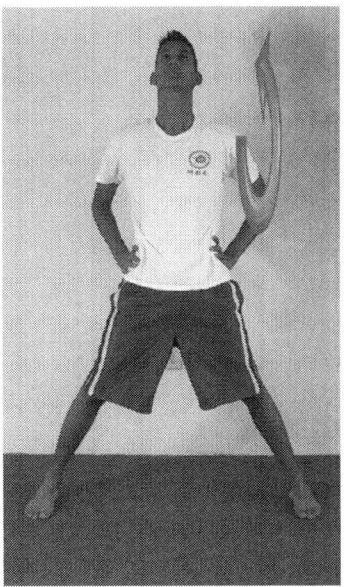

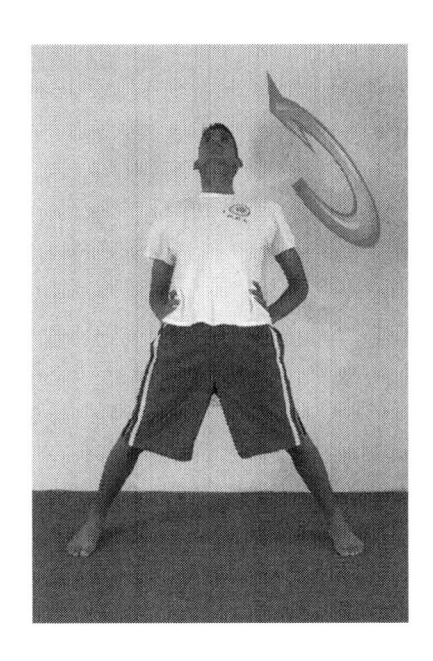

FLOOR (SITTING) STRETCHES

You have now completed the upper body stretches and are ready to move on to the floor stretches.

SITTING LEG STRETCHES

Begin by sitting on the floor, extend your left leg straight forward and cross your right leg on top of your left thigh. Hold your right ankle with your right hand while gently rotating your right ankle with your left hand. Do this rotation in both directions.

Sitting Ankle-Leg Stretches - ...then Switch Legs/Ankles

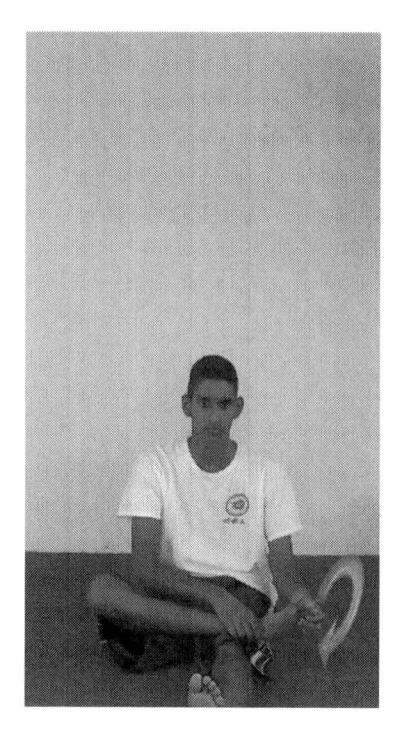

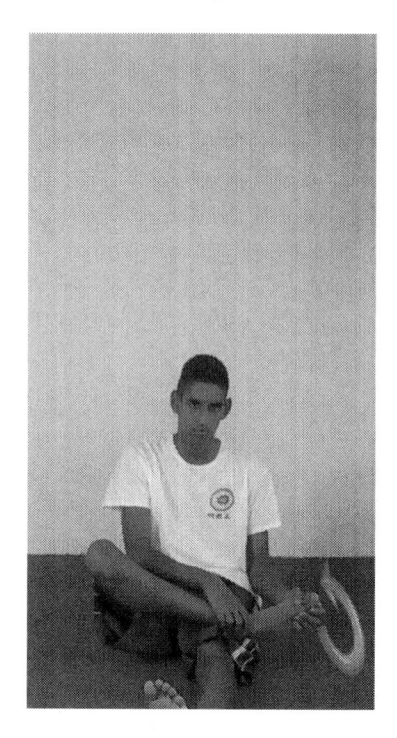

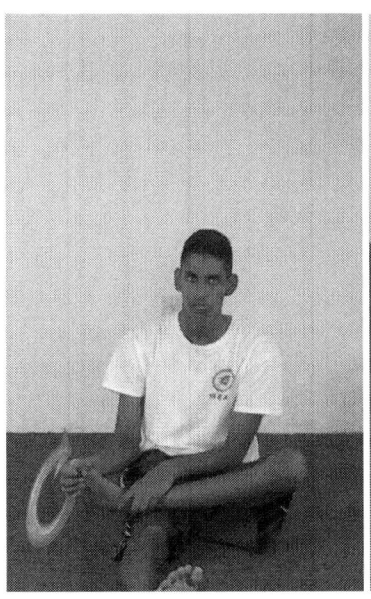

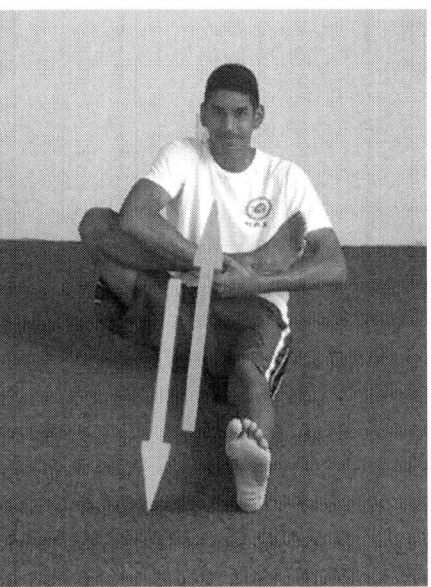

When finished, grab your right foot and ankle with both hands and bring them as close to your chest as possible. Hold for a few seconds, and kick out that right leg in the air two or three times. Now, switch and do the same with the left leg and ankle, using the right hand. Follow up with raising the left foot and ankle to the chest, and kick out the left leg after bringing to the chest.

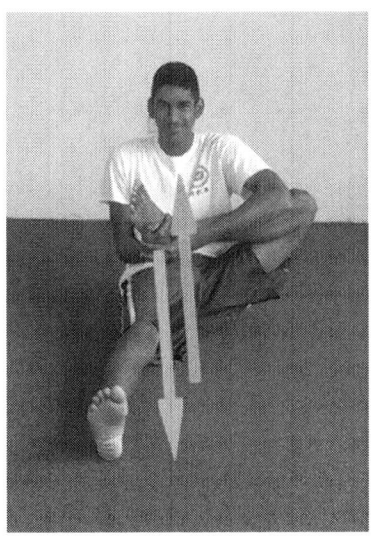

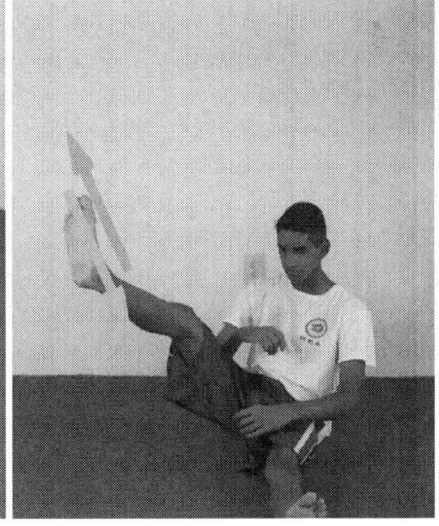

Now you are going to reach for and grab the bottom of your right foot from the <u>inside</u> with your right thumb down pointing down to the floor. Gently lift your right leg straight up, holding your foot, and stretch that leg as far as your arm will allow. Bend the leg inward, bringing the ankle and foot to your body as far in as you can, and repeat the stretch straight upward. Do this stretch two times. Now, continue to hold the same right foot with the right hand, and stretch the leg out to the right side as far as you can, leaving the extended left leg straight out without changing its position (next page). Do this outside right leg stretch two times. When finished, kick out the leg a couple of times. Then repeat the same stretch with the left leg in the same manner, using the left hand to grab the left foot from the <u>inside</u>, thumb down, stretching upward and to the left side, and kick out the left leg when finished.

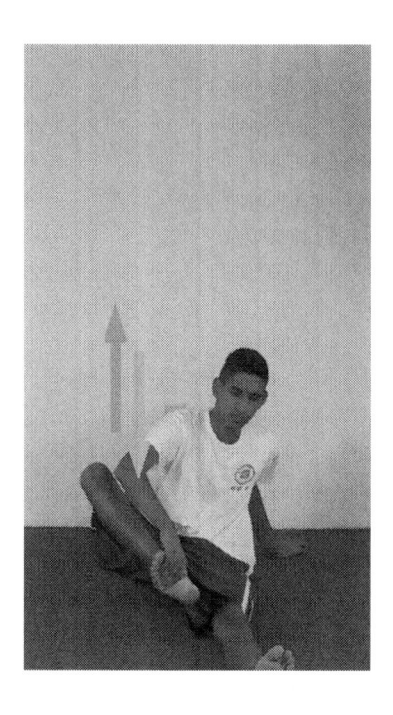

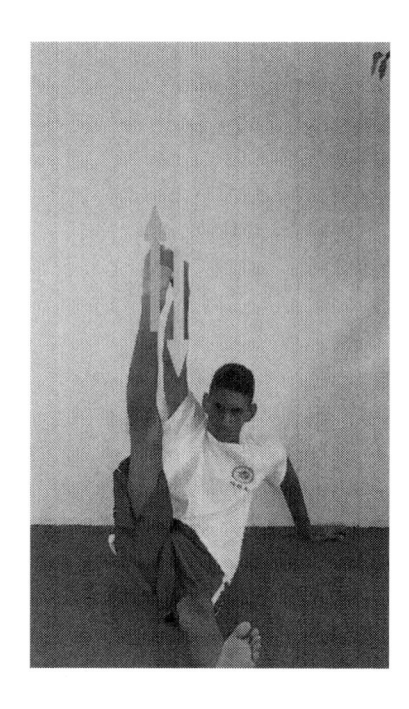

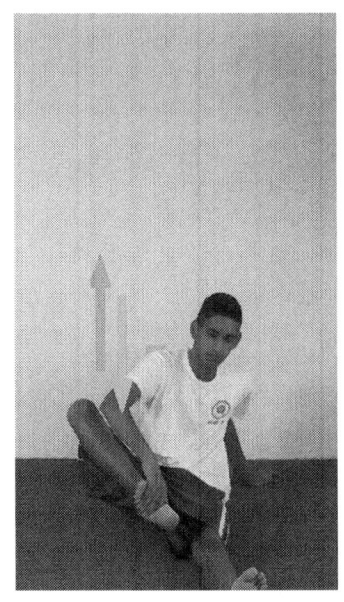

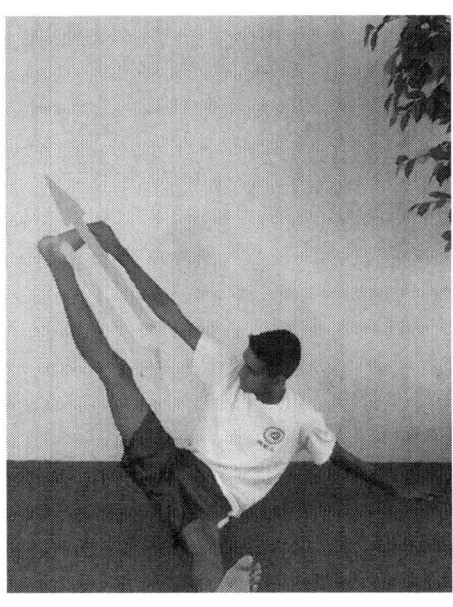

Then Shake Leg and Switch - Raising Leg Stretches - Front and Side

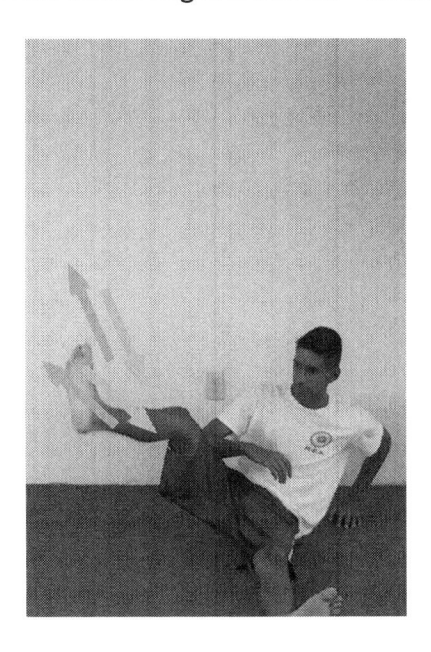

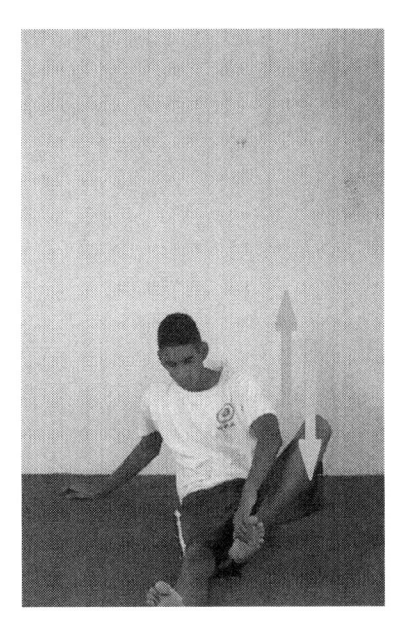

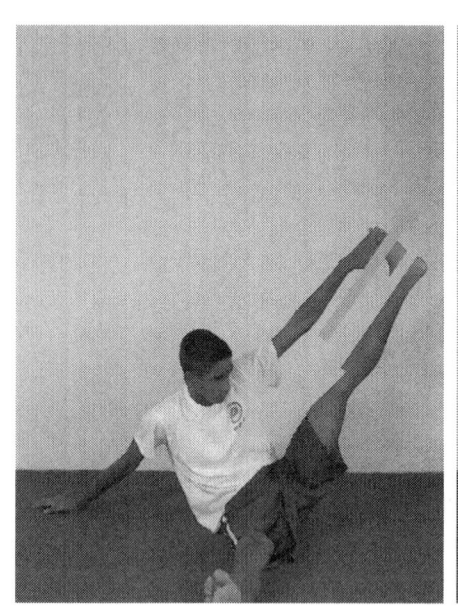

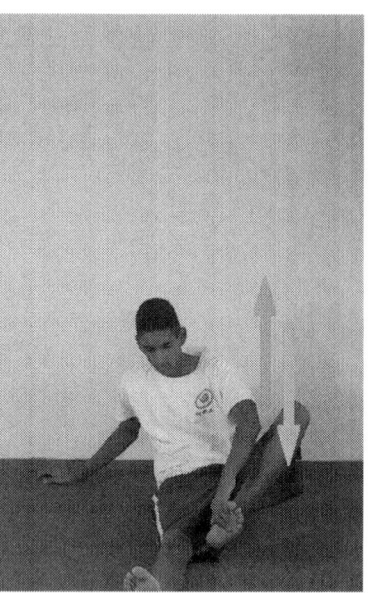

...and Shake this Leg

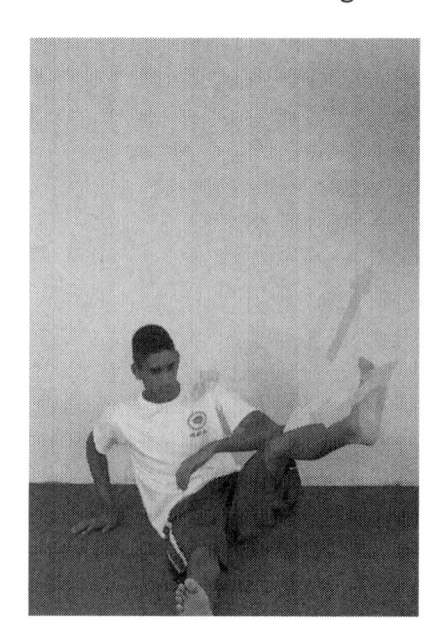

Now we are ready to stretch both legs while sitting on the floor. Open your legs as wide as comfortable. Initially you may not be able to spread your legs very wide. Don't worry about this. You want to begin safely, only spreading your legs to where you feel a small tug on them when stretching. In time you will be able to spread your legs wider for a better stretch. Don't be discouraged if you cannot open your legs as wide as you wish. Some people's skeleton systems may not allow for a total, straight line stretch. You don't need an exact straight line sideways stretch to gain the benefits of the stretch. Also, you do not want to force this stretch because an injury from forcing the stretch like a torn ligament or tendon will take a long time to heal, and can be very painful. Therefore, begin your stretch slowly, and work on making your stretch bigger with time the more you stretch.

BREATHING AND STRETCHING

Breathing Tip Reminder:

When you bend forward try to first inhale before you bend, then exhale when bending into the stretch. When you transition to the next stretch, again inhale when leaving the earlier stretch, and exhale when reaching for the next stretch. **For brevity, I will not repeat this tip with each exercise description, but try to remember to follow it particularly when doing the following stretches. This suggestion also applies to other stretching exercises.**

Your first stretch with legs extended will be to bend forward. If you can place your chest on the floor without pain or extreme discomfort, you can do so. You can place your hands or arms on the floor if possible. Again, do not force this stretch. After bending forward, sit upright and bend to the right side, reaching for the right ankle. After grabbing your right ankle with both hands, and holding for a few seconds, return to the upright position and continue bending to the left, reaching for the left ankle. Hold for a few seconds and again return to the center in an upright position. Bend forward again as far as you can. If you can, when you bend forward, try grabbing your toes with your hands as you bend forward.

SITTING TRUNK & OPEN LEG/BACK STRETCHES

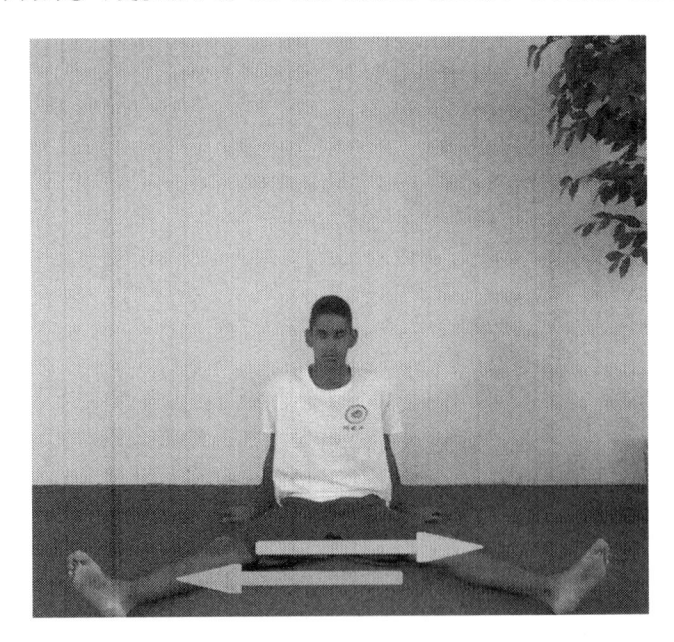

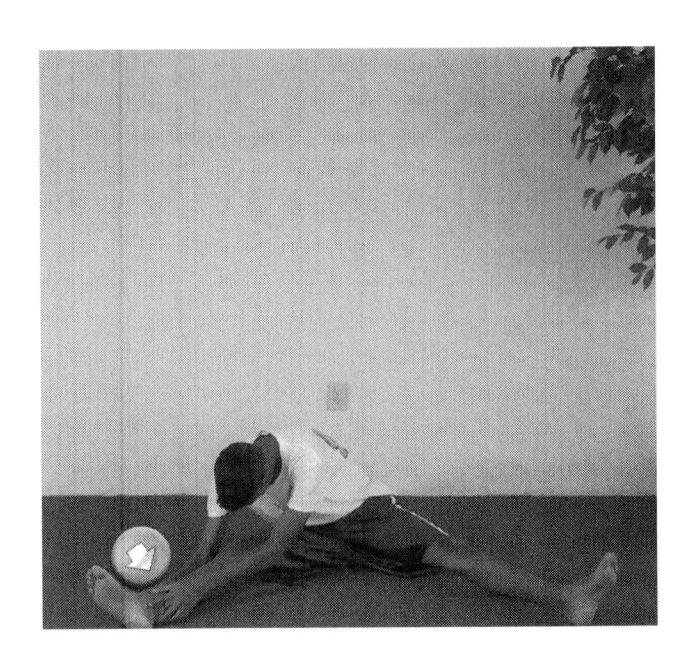

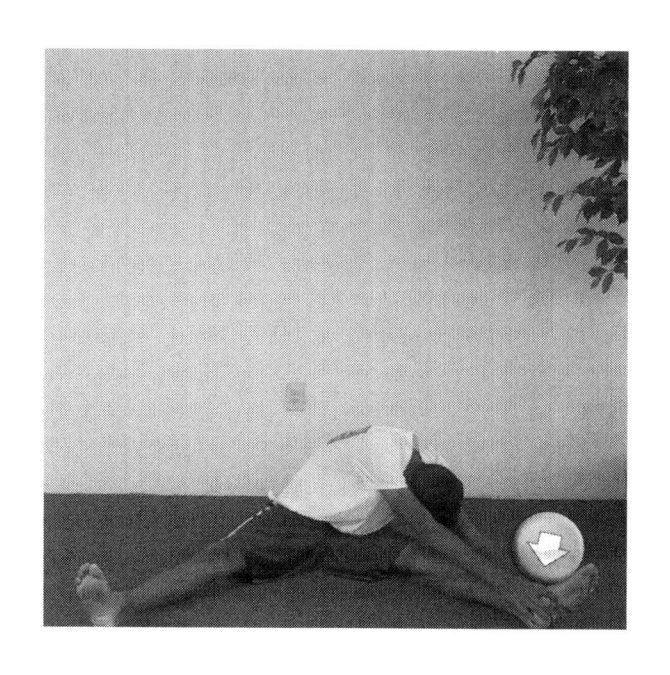

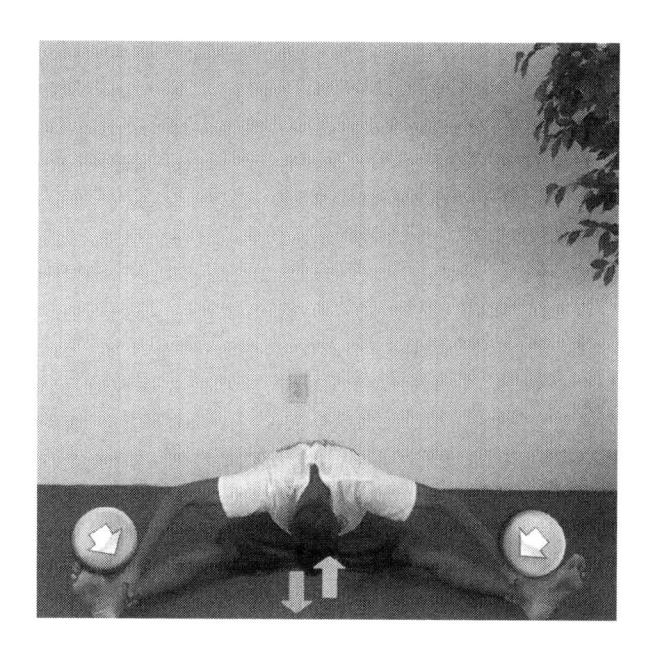

At this stage, it is helpful to warm up the thigh muscles specifically by thumping the inside, top and outside of the leg thigh muscles with your fists. You will want to thump these large muscles hard enough to work the muscle from the knee to the groin and in both directions, but not too hard as to cause discomfort or bruising. This type of massage works the muscle tissue and encourages more blood flow to the muscle.

Striking the Back of Thigh Muscle (outside upper leg)

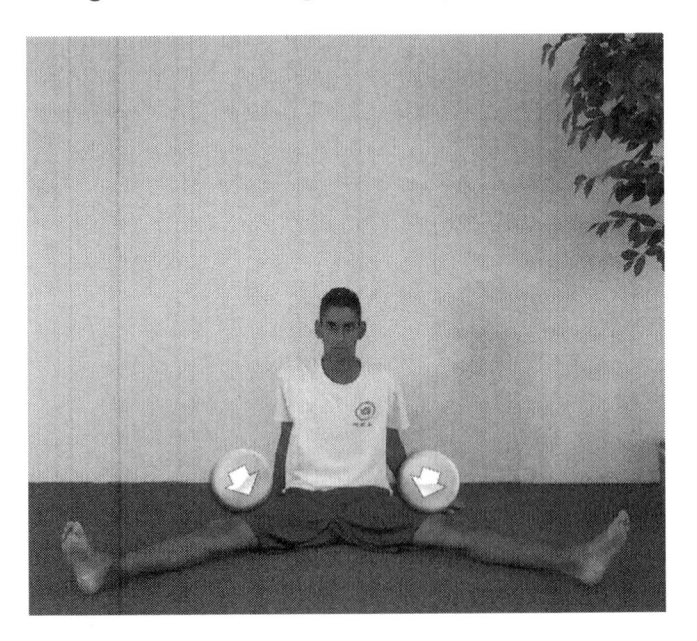

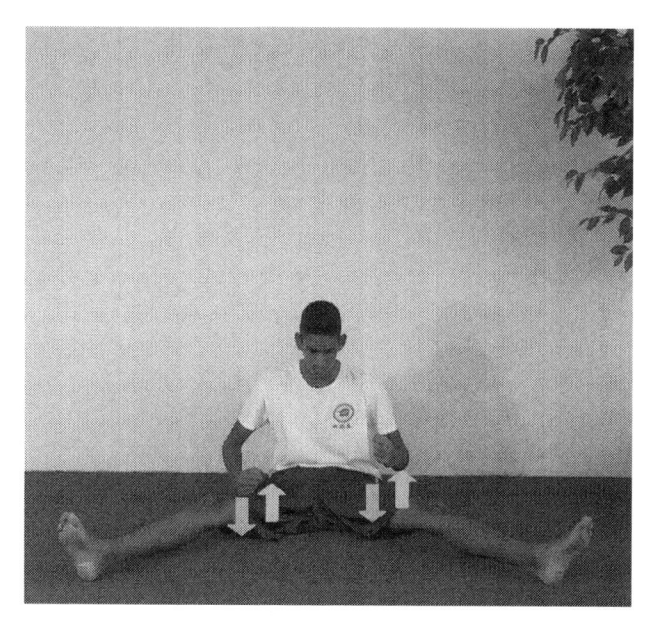

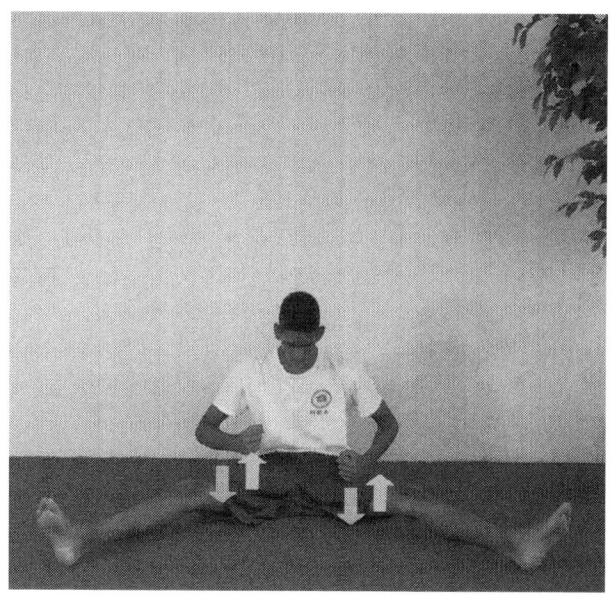

Striking Top of Thigh

Striking Inside of Thigh

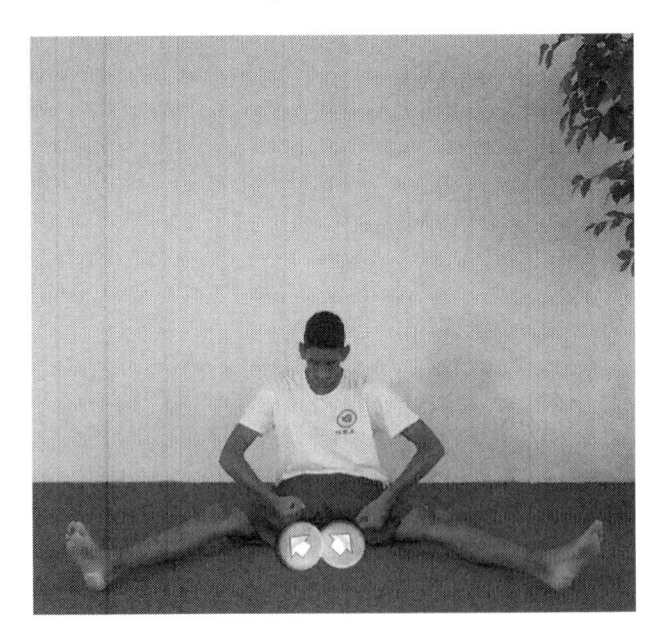

Striking Outside of Thigh

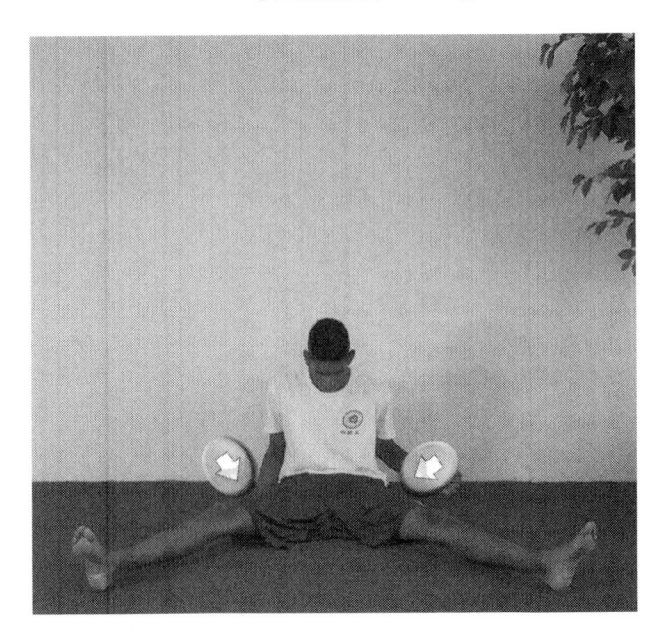

...and Repeat Top, Inside & Outside Striking the Thigh 2-3 times

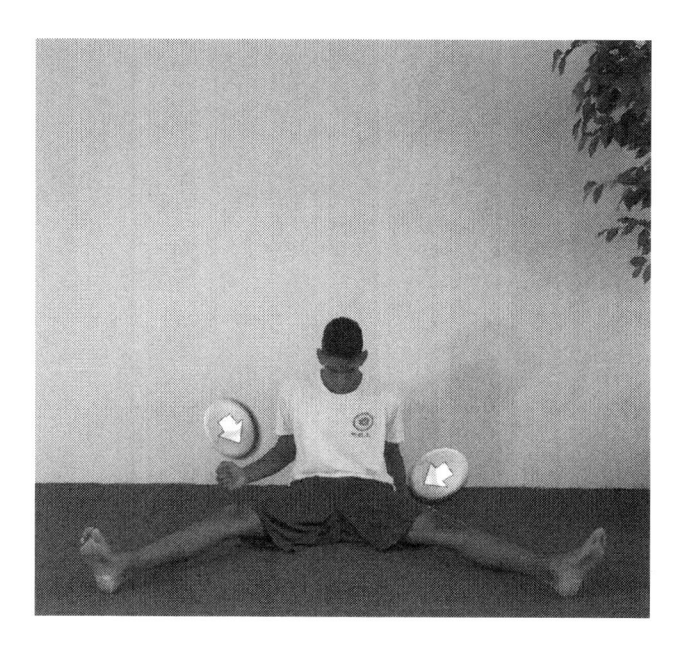

When completing this leg thigh muscle preparation, try to open your legs a little further, and repeat the same left and right stretches you did earlier, and this time place your <u>head on your knee</u> with each left and right stretch. Do this same stretch again while reaching around the <u>bottom of the foot</u> with each hand for an even better stretch.

Now bring your legs together, extending them straight out in front of you and shake your legs gently. With your knees "locked" down and leg straight, first inhale and then bend down and grab your ankles while exhaling. Sit up again while inhaling, and grab your ankles once again while exhaling. Finally, do the same stretch, this time grabbing around the bottom of both feet with your respective right and left hand and place your head on your knees. Hold this stretch for a few seconds and return to the upright position. Again, shake out your legs.

Sitting Front Leg Stretch - Begin with Ankle Touch

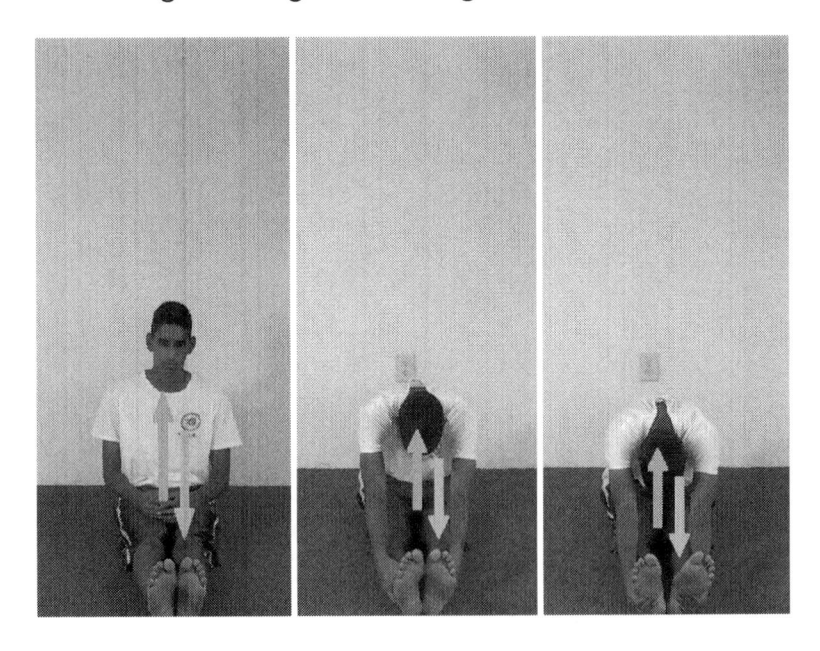

...then Same Stretch - Ankle Touch with Head on Knee

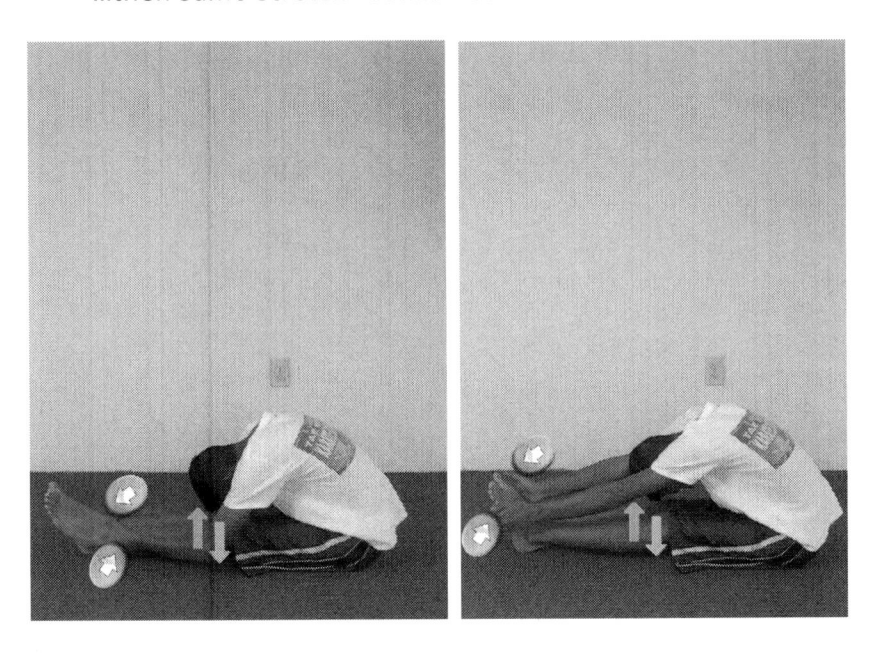

...then Toe Touch with Head on Knee

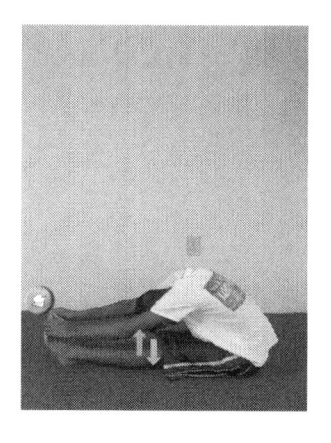

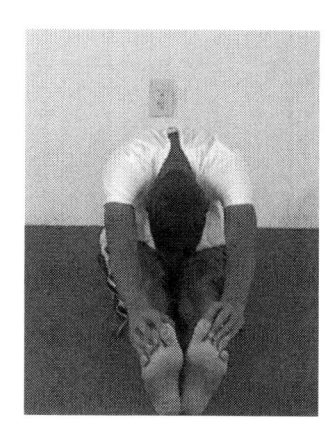

If you are flexible enough, with legs wide, point your toes to the ceiling and fold your arms in front of your chest while looking sitting upright. Next, try to place your chest on the floor and spread your arms toward your feet. Do NOT force the stretch. Tip: It helps to turn your head to either side for maximum stretch and results.

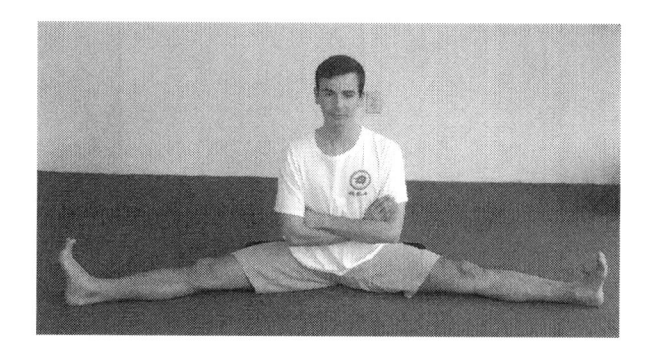

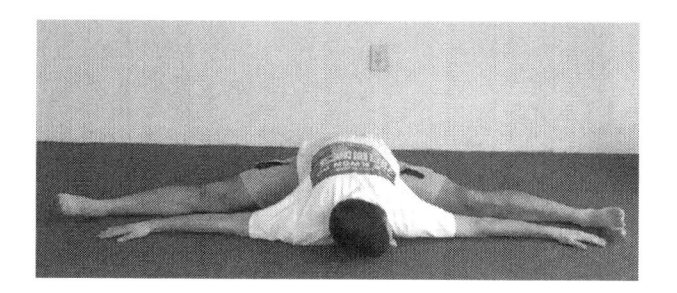

Sitting on the floor, bring your legs now into a "butterfly position" (next page). The butterfly position is made by bending your legs and bringing your feet together, sole to sole, and holding both feet together with your hands. After inhaling, bend forward while exhaling and place your head on your toes, or as close to your toes as possible, without undue discomfort. Do not force the stretch. Hold a few seconds, sit up and repeat. You can do this stretch two or three times. After the final stretch, take your hands and gently push your knees to the floor. Again, be careful not to push your knees down too hard, too fast, or too far to avoid unnecessary injury. It is **not** important that you push your knees to the floor, only that you get a good stretch. When finished extend both legs straight out in front of you and shake out both legs well.

Butterfly Stretch - Repeat sequence 3 times, pull in feet more each time

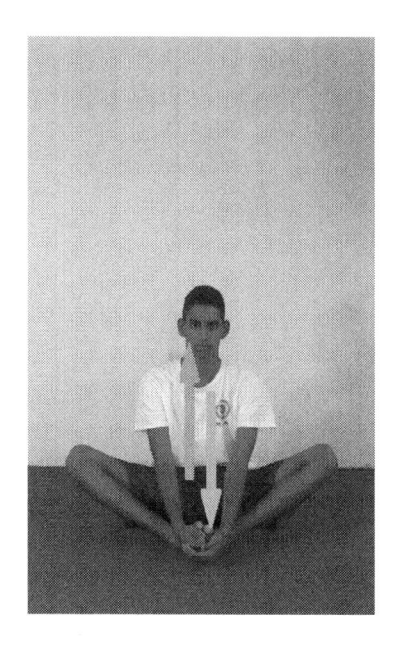

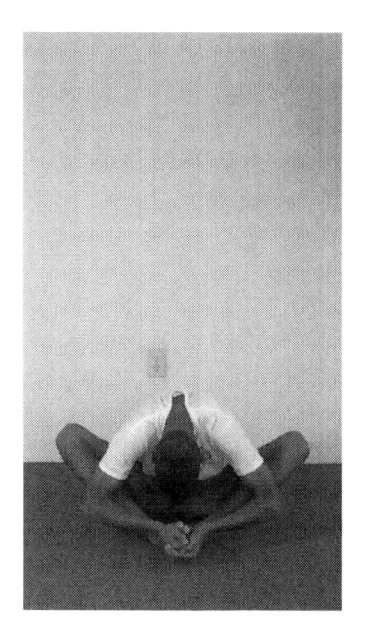

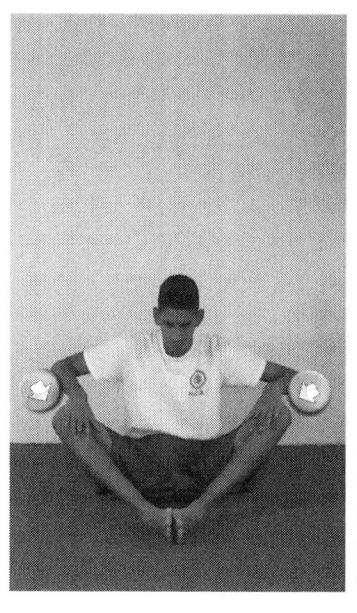

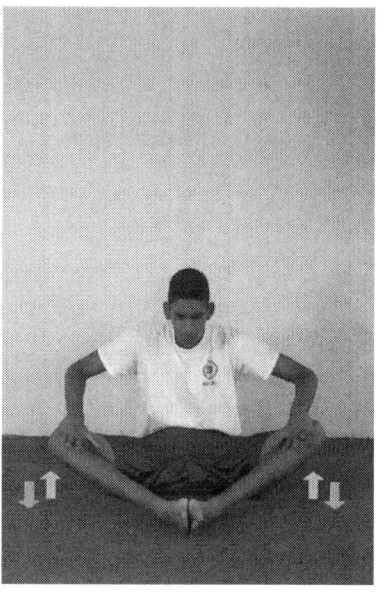

SITTING TRUNK & BACK STRETCHES (ROLL BACKS)

While sitting with legs fully extended forward, using your legs roll backward onto your shoulders. It is important that you try to place your body weight on your shoulders and not on your middle back.

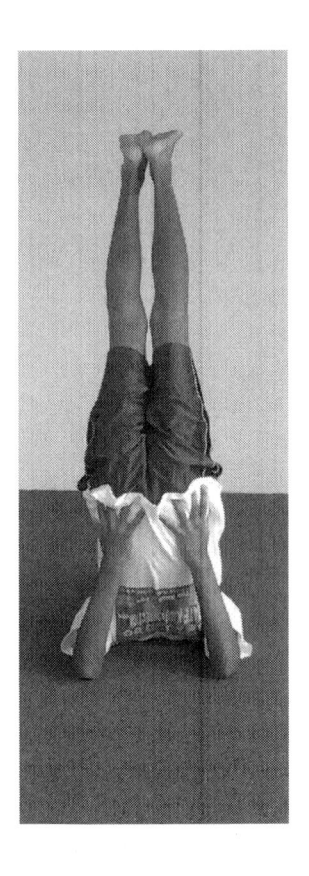

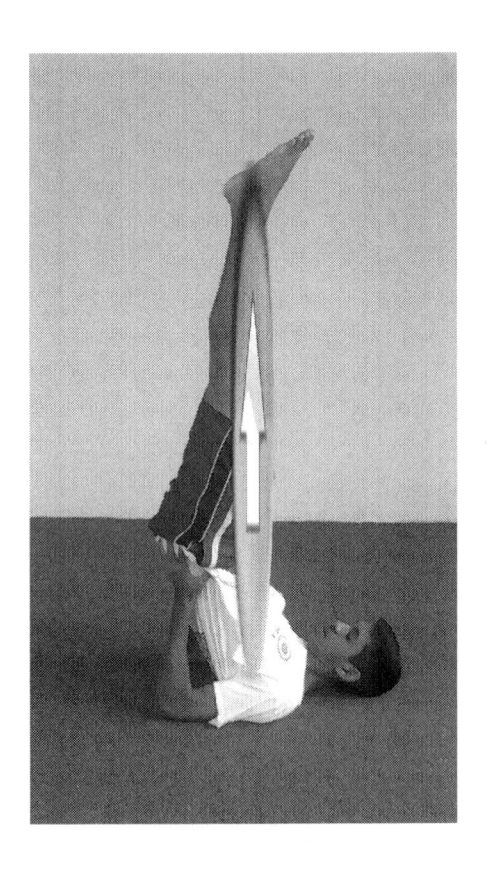

To do this you will need to place your hands on your lower back while supporting your body with your elbows placed firmly on the floor (see above). Keep your elbows on the floor and the palms of your hands on your lower back while extending your legs straight upward, making an imaginary straight line from your shoulders to your ankles, legs/ankles touching, toes pointing upward toward the ceiling as far as possible.

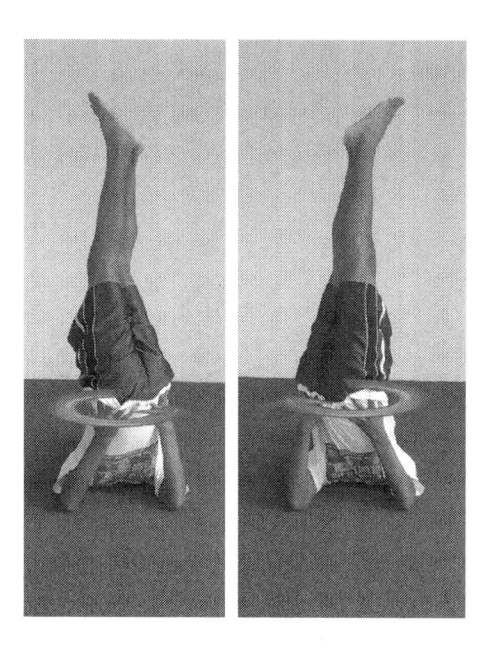

With toes pointed upward, twist your trunk (waist) to the right and to the left as far as possible, and repeat two or three times. Then <u>open</u> your legs, and while leaving them open, repeat twisting your waist with legs extended in both directions.

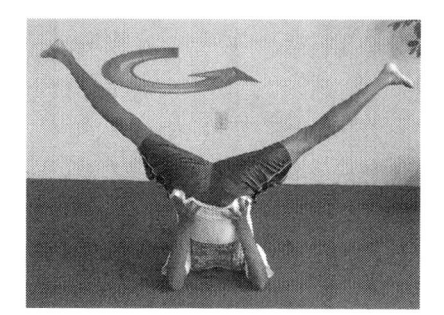

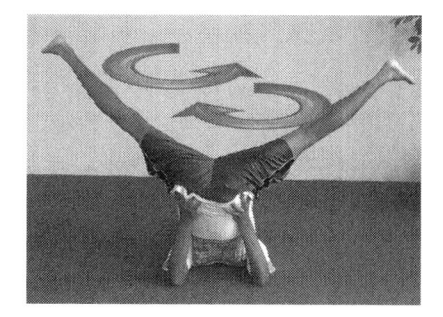

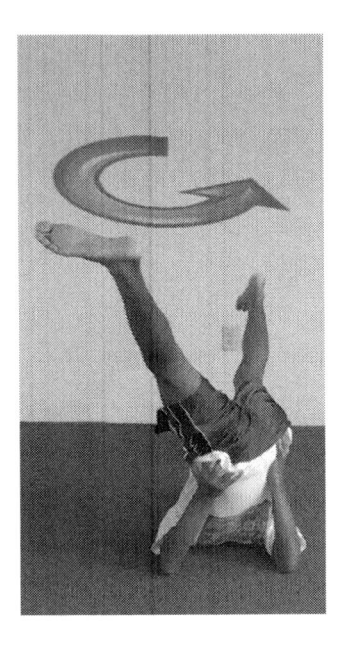

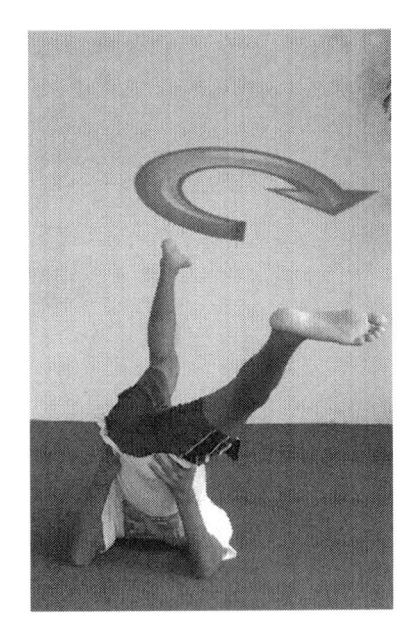

Return your legs to the upright position with ankles touching, bring your toes pointed down (back) toward your knees, and move your legs in a forward bicycling movement for approximately 4 or 5 rotations.

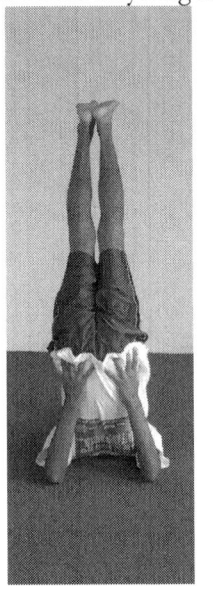

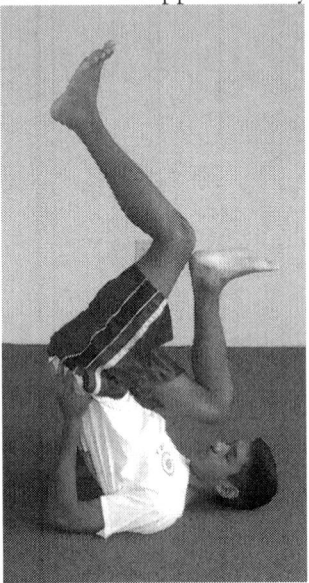

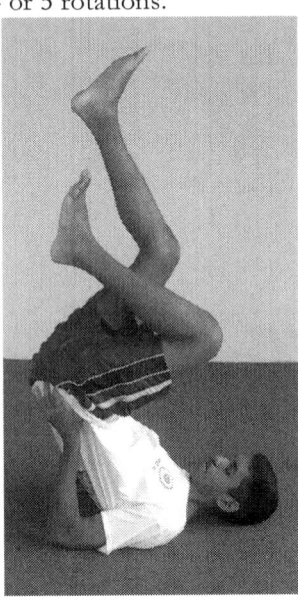

Reverse the bicycling movement for 4-5 rotations. With legs returned to the upright position and toes pointed to the ceiling. If you wish, you can repeat the left/right twisting movements once or twice to finish the exercise.

The next and final stretch in this series of waist/leg exercises requires more flexibility and requires greater care of the neck. Beginners might want to skip this exercise until they become more flexible in general, and have more confidence of their stretching limits.

IMPORTANT NOTE: It is recommended that **ALL** readers discuss this neck/leg stretch first with a doctor or qualified physical therapist to see if it presents any degree of unnecessary risk. Readers with any experienced or suspected neck problems should avoid this exercise until discussing with their doctors. It is not necessary to do this specific stretch to receive the benefits of the other stretching exercises previously described.

For those readers able to proceed with this specific exercise, to add an additional challenge, while supporting your body on your shoulders, feet pointed upward toward the ceiling, you will carefully and slowly lower your feet over your head while lowering your legs to touch your toes to the floor behind your head with legs open wide (see next page).

NOTE: It is important that the reader relax the neck as much as possible, and <u>AVOID ANY FORCED EXTENSION OF THE NECK</u>, as described earlier in this book on neck circle exercises.

Once again, with the body resting on the shoulders, hands supporting the lower back and legs open wide, <u>**after making a deliberate effort to relax your neck muscles**</u>, allow your legs **s-l-o-w-l-y** to lower to the floor. If you are having no discomfort or pain, you can attempt to touch your toes to the floor for a couple of seconds, and return to the upright seated position, legs straight ahead in front of you, ankles together as you slowly bend forward to touch your toes with both hands once again. Allow your entire body to relax as much as possible throughout this entire exercise.

NOTE: It is NOT necessary to touch the floor to receive a benefit from this stretch, particularly if there is any significant discomfort or pain experienced while attempting this stretch.

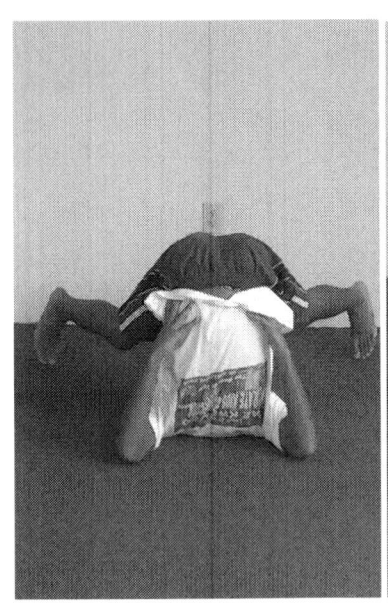

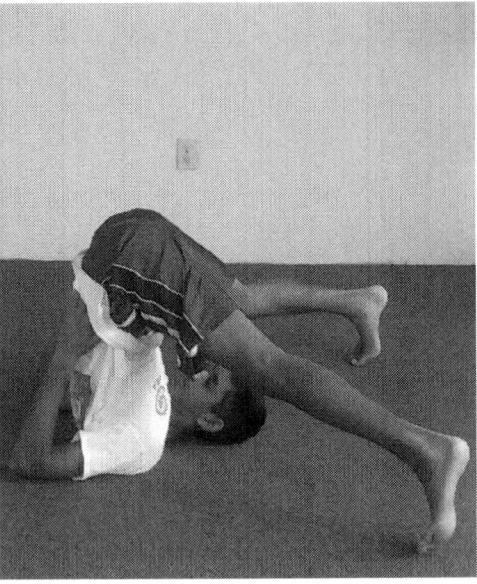

Now you can return to the sitting position on the floor by lowering your legs straight out in front of you, and shake out both legs. This segment of stretching is completed with you inhaling and exhaling as you bend forward, sitting, legs/knees "locked," and grab your ankles with both hands, head on your knees. Now you can sit up again, inhale and exhale.

The next back stretch is to strengthen your lower back (see next page). Turn onto your stomach and place your hands aside your shoulders. Push with both hands, raising your shoulders and chest off the floor, tilting your head back as far as comfortably possible. Remember not to extend your head backward with force or to push too hard to avoid hyperextension of the neck. The neck is very fragile with tiny bones, and you will want to protect it by gently easing it back, as you look toward the ceiling. When you raise your chest (upper half of your body), inhale. When you are in the raised position, exhale, relax, and stay up for a few seconds, and return to the beginning position. Repeat this lower back stretch two or three times. When finished, raise your body, cross your feet, sit back placing your seat on your heels, forehead on the floor, and your arms straight out on the floor, overlapping one hand over the other, as if to make an "arrowhead" with the hands, and enjoy the stretch.

On Stomach Back-Neck Stretch

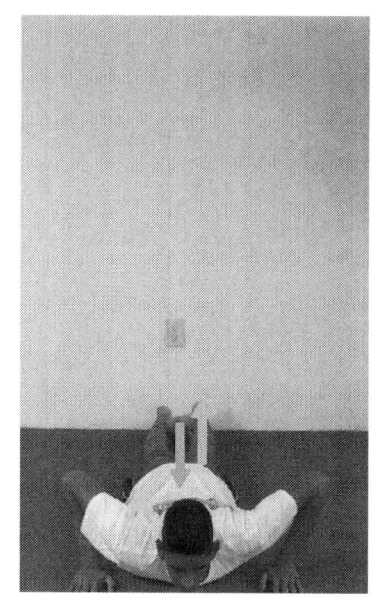

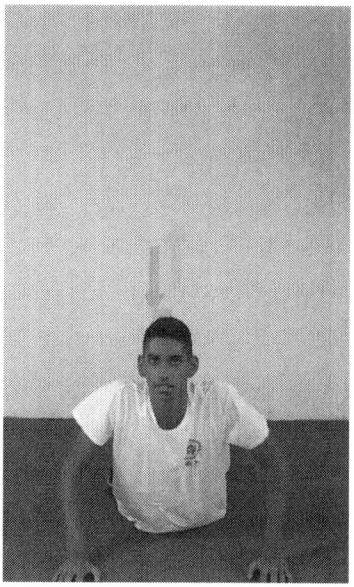

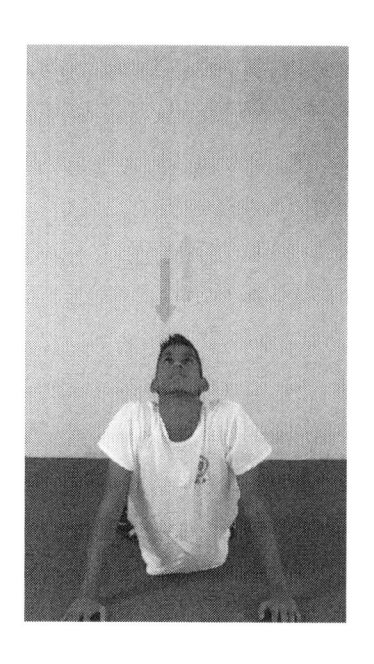

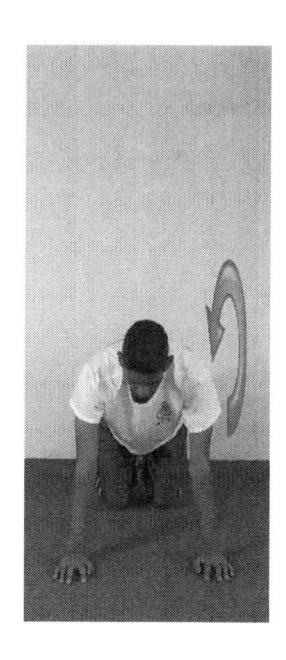

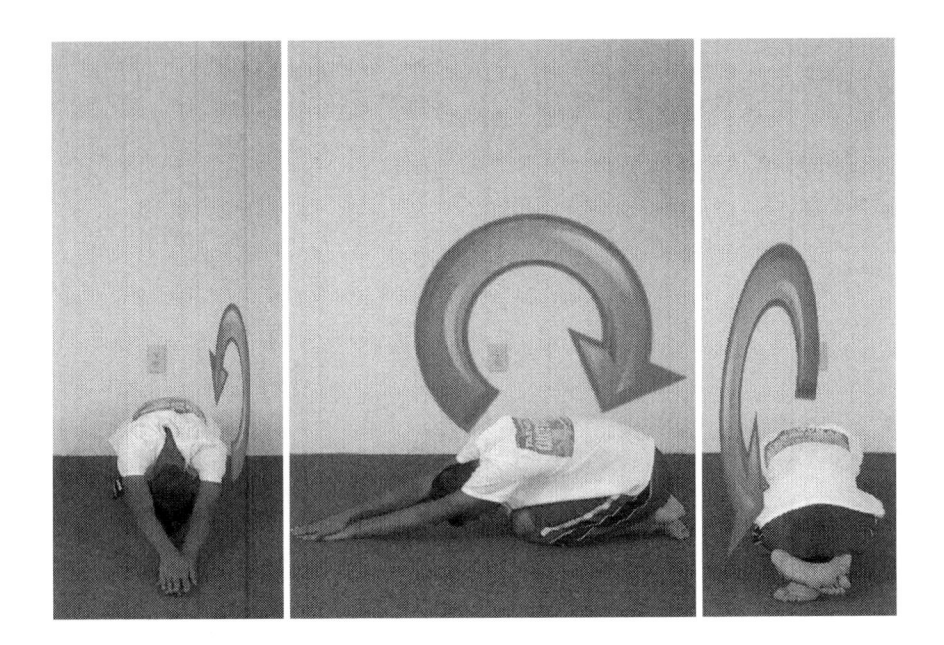

PARTNER STRETCHES

SITTING PARTNER STRETCHES

The following partner stretches are best done with a partner if one is available. The first partner stretch is called an open leg stretch. If you do not have a partner to work out with, you can use the wall or a piece of furniture to assist you with the stretch.

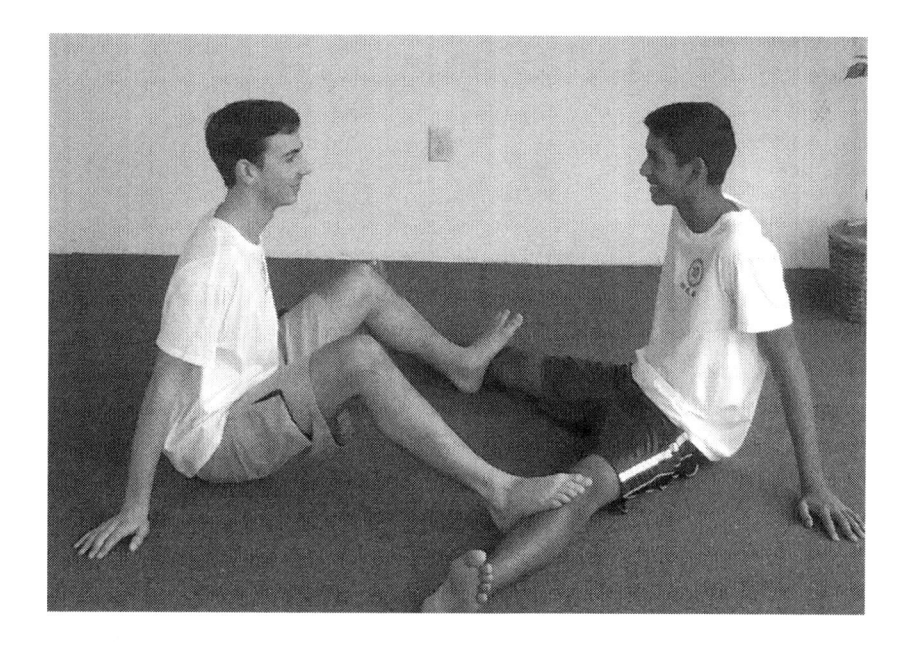

For this stretch, sit on the floor facing your partner (or the wall, sofa, etc.) You will take turns stretching each other. With your partner facing you, legs spread apart, place your feet about 5-8 inches directly below your partner's knees. NOTE: Do NOT place your feet lower on your partner's leg to avoid stressing the knee joints.

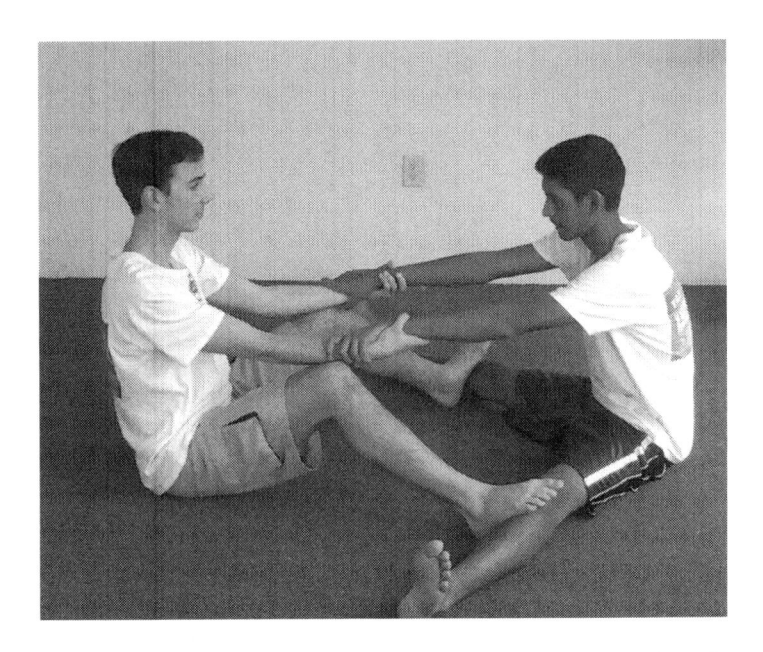

Grab your partner's wrists or you can grab each other's wrists for more support. With your feet placed slightly below your partner's knee, gently pull your partner forward until your partner "taps" your arm. Tapping lets you know your partner has stretched far enough for this stretch and you should return your partner to their original upright sitting position.

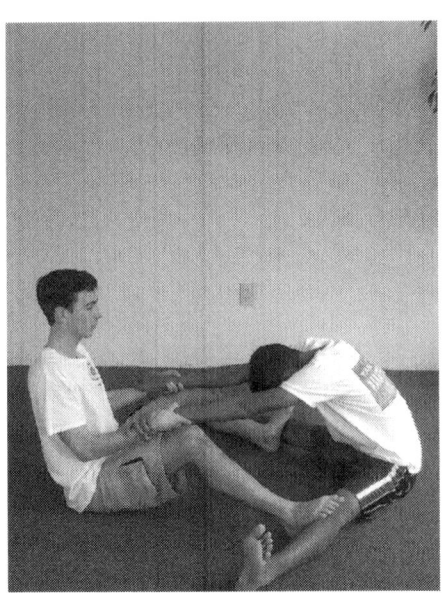

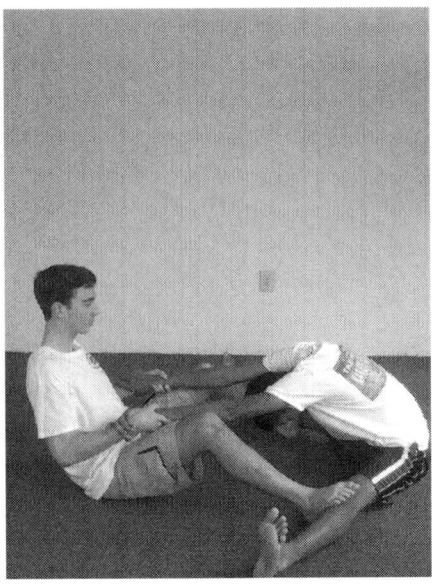

It is very important and needs to be stressed here that partners should <u>pay close attention to and honor their partner's tap</u>, slowly returning to the original upright position to avoid a groin injury. This type of injury is very painful, and can take much time to heal. With practice and experience, you and your partner can predict how much to challenge this stretch for the best, but safe, results. Do this stretch for your partner two or three times. If your partner is already quite flexible and has a good stretch, you also can grab your partner's elbows and have your partner do the same to you to provide a bigger, more beneficial stretch. Once you have stretched out your partner, it is your turn for your partner to help you with this stretch, using the same procedure and guidelines.

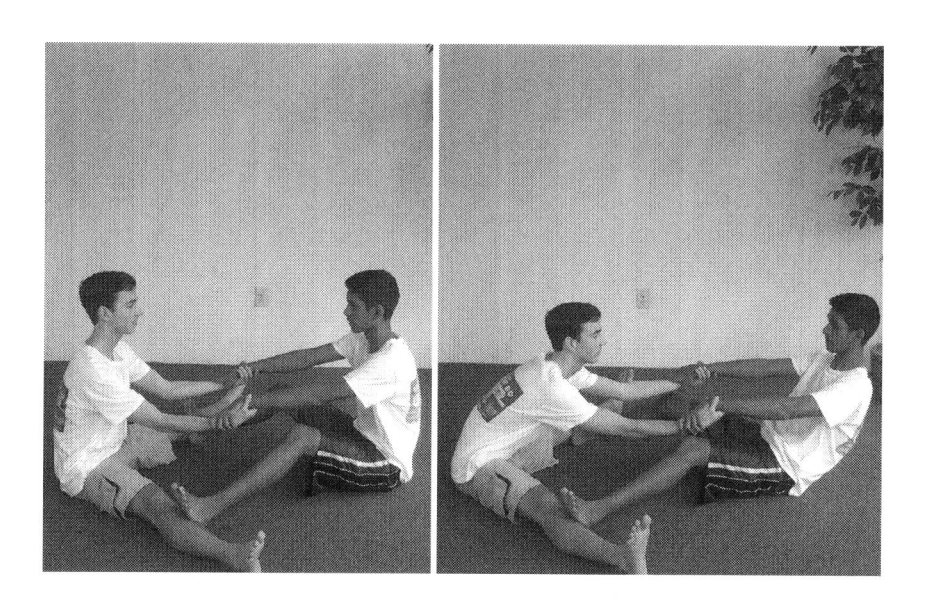

If your partner is very flexible and has an exceptionally good stretch, try grabbing behind your partner's elbows (see next page.) This will allow you to apply more stretch as you lean backwards. Again, be sure to go slowly and attend to your partner's tap, indicating you need to relax the stretch and slowly pause or return to the starting position.

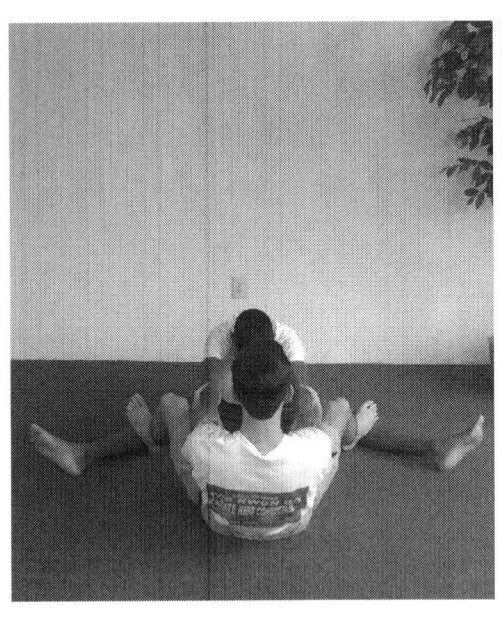

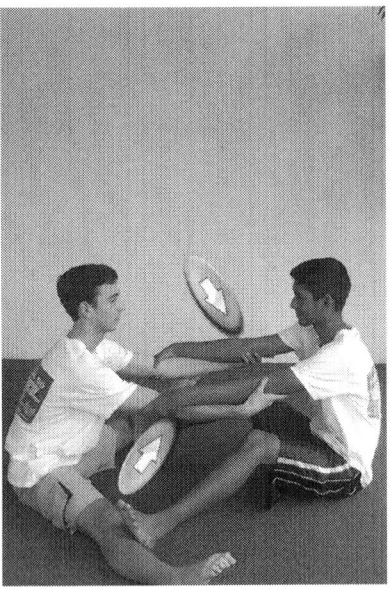

If you have no partner, you can still benefit from this stretch by sitting, facing the wall, legs spread and feet against the wall, by taking your hands to push your center (hips) as close (forward) to the wall as possible, and hold for a few seconds. You can do this several times for maximum benefit. Again, be careful and mindful of all safety concerns while using this stretch.

STRENGTH EXERCISES

If you want to extend your flexibility and stretching routine, you can proceed to more strength-building exercises, such as push-ups and sit-ups. Most people are familiar with push-ups and sit-ups even if they don't include them in their exercise or stretching workouts.

PUSH-UPS

When doing push-ups, beginners should start with their hands flat on the floor, placed beneath and slightly wider than the shoulders, chest/shoulders in the "up" position, and the balls of the feet making direct contact with the floor. This is called the starting position. There should be an imaginary straight line from the ankles to the shoulders, so that there is no sagging of the body's mid-section. With head slightly raised and looking straight forward, begin your push-up by lowering your chest toward the floor, allowing your elbows to bend. Once your chest lowers to approximately 4-5 inches from the floor, begin pushing your chest back up to starting position. Repeat this movement as many times as you can comfortably perform the entire downward and upward movement. As you become more experienced and stronger, you will be able to challenge yourself to do more and more push-ups which will make you even stronger. This is an excellent exercise for building the pectorals, deltoids and triceps muscles.

Strength Exercises - Pushups using <u>Flat Palms</u> for Support

Begin your pushup in the "up" position on palms or knuckles, as shown:

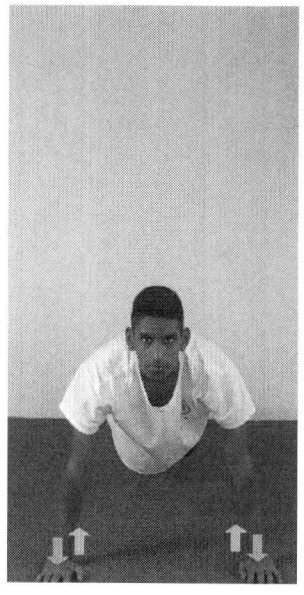

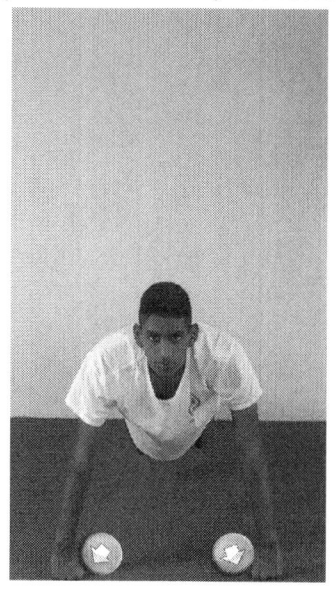

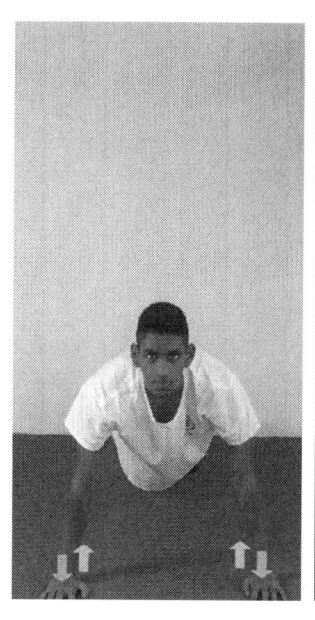

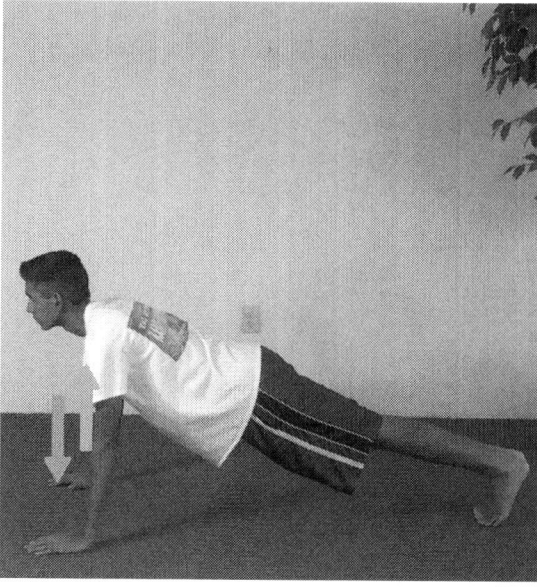

69

Lower Your Body to the Lower Position, and Return to Starting position

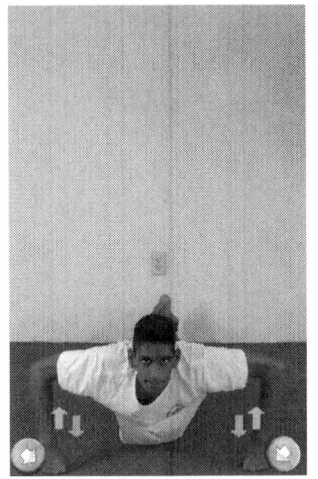

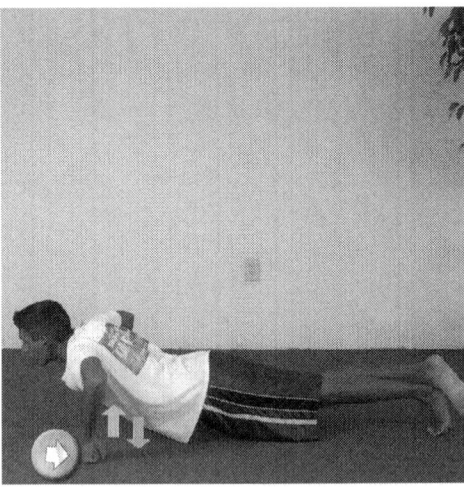

KNUCKLE PUSH-UPS (ADVANCED EXERCISE)

Once you become stronger and more experienced doing regular push-ups, you can challenge yourself by doing them on your knuckles. These are advanced push-up exercises. The form and procedure remains the same except that you begin by making a fist and support your chest/shoulders on your "contact knuckles." You will recall that the contact knuckles are the first two knuckles next to the thumbs, namely your pointer and middle finger knuckles. This is the part of the fist which makes "contact" with a target when used for striking. Martial art students do "knuckle push-ups" for two primary reasons: first, to build up calluses on their contact knuckles for punching and board breaking, as well as to strengthen the wrists for similar contact when breaking or sparring (fighting.) If it hurts when you first try doing knuckle push-ups, do only a few and build up strength and endurance as you gain more experience and tolerance. If you decide to accept this challenge, be sure to keep your wrists strong during these push-ups to avoid your wrist collapsing during the exercise and spraining the wrist.

Advanced Alternate Pushups - Advanced participants <u>on Knuckles</u>

(Strengthens the Wrists and creates calluses on the knuckles)

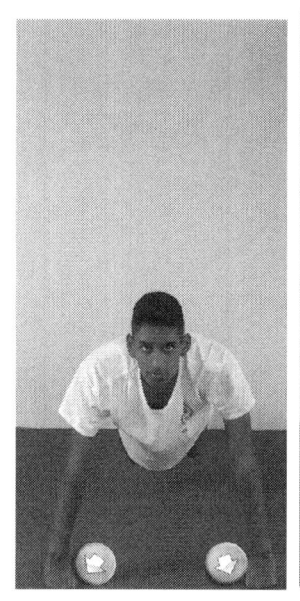

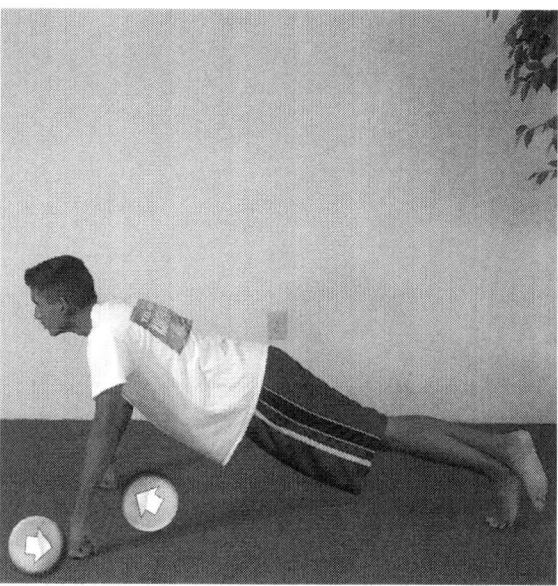

ONE-ARM PUSH-UPS

There are also one-arm pushups (next page) also which begin in much the same way. One-arm push-ups are usually done with one hand flat on the ground, legs spread wide, and the other arm placed behind and on the back.

As with the regular two arm push-ups, you lower your body using only one arm to within 4-5 inches of the floor, and push up to the starting position. Do as many of these exercises as you can safely do, challenging yourself more and more as you become stronger and more experienced.

Note: this is a very challenging but optional exercise, and should only be attempted by those students who are experienced doing regular push-ups to avoid injuries to the face, especially the nose, mouth and teeth.

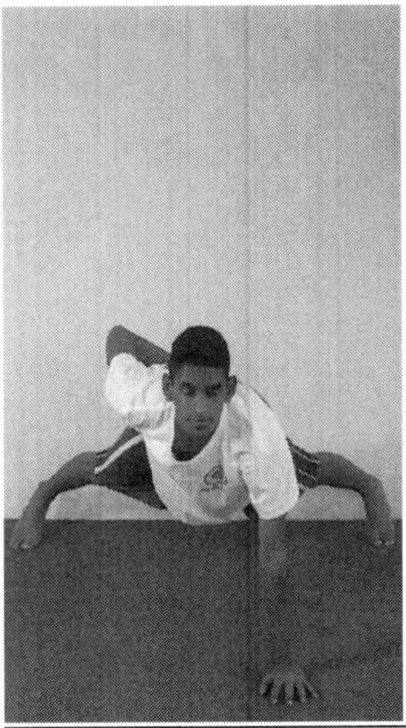
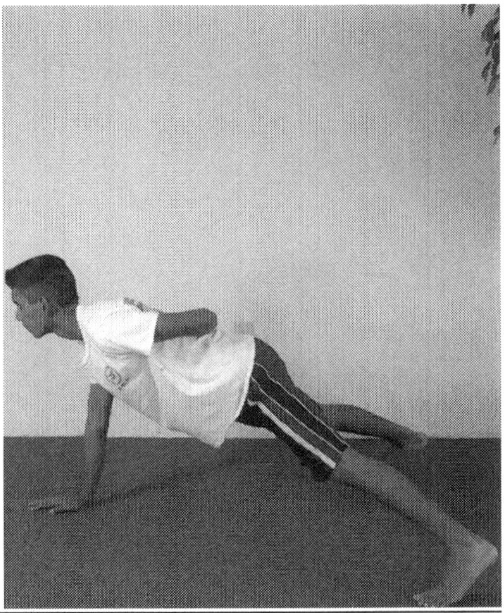
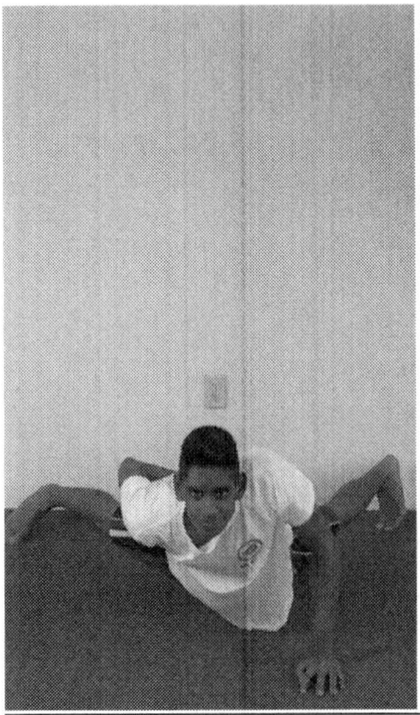
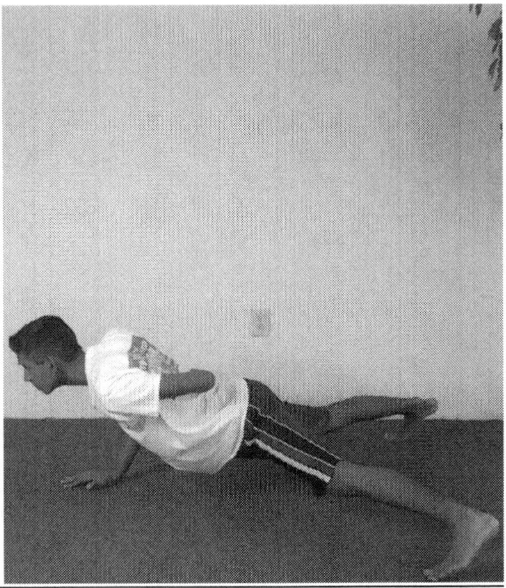

PARTNER PUSH-UPS

If you have a partner, you can add an additional challenge to your push-up exercises. Have your partner kneel and assume an "all-fours" position, supporting the body on both hands and both knees. You will assume the usual original push-up position (with hands flat on the floor or on knuckles - your choice) directly in front of your partner. Now place your shins (the part of your leg between your knee and your ankle) on each side of your partner's head, resting your shins on your partner's back and shoulders.

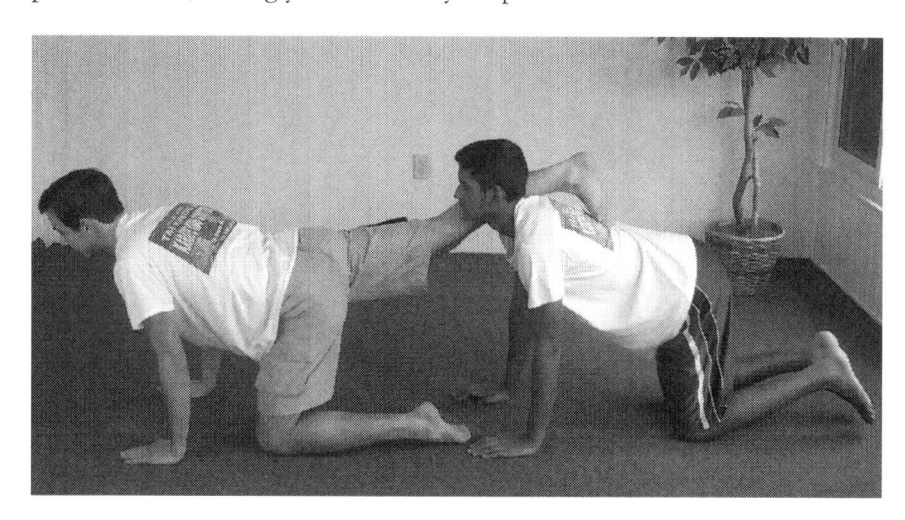

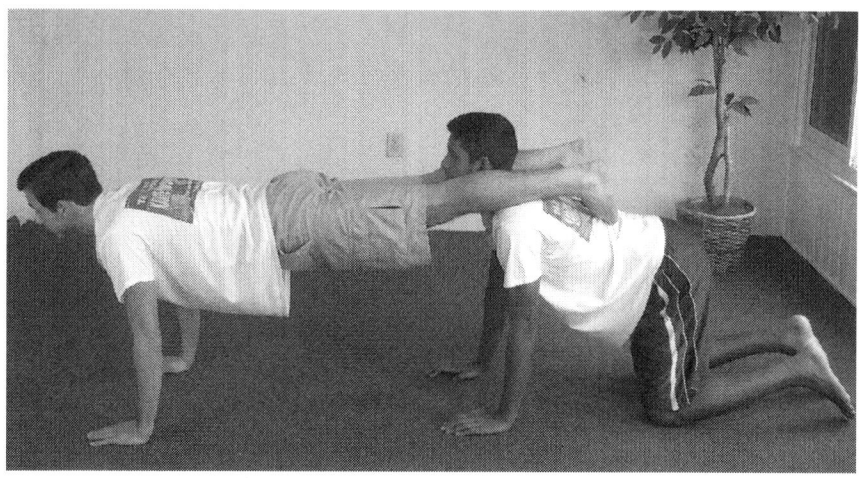

Begin to do your own push-ups with your legs supported by your partner's shoulders, while your partner remains still. Lower your body within a few inches of the floor and return to the starting position, and repeat as many push-ups as desirable. Only the front partner does the push-ups.

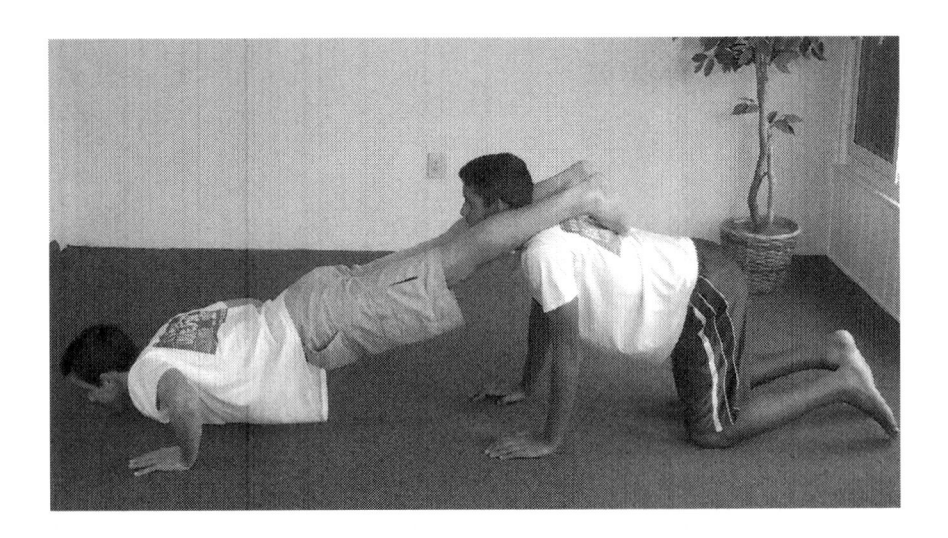

The next challenge is for your partner to assume the usual, inclined push-up position, while your body is parallel to the floor (straight across) as you support your upper body with your hands and arms and your lower body with your shins on your partner's back. You now can begin to do your own push-ups while your partner remains still. To increase the challenge, both of you can do your push-ups simultaneously (next page).

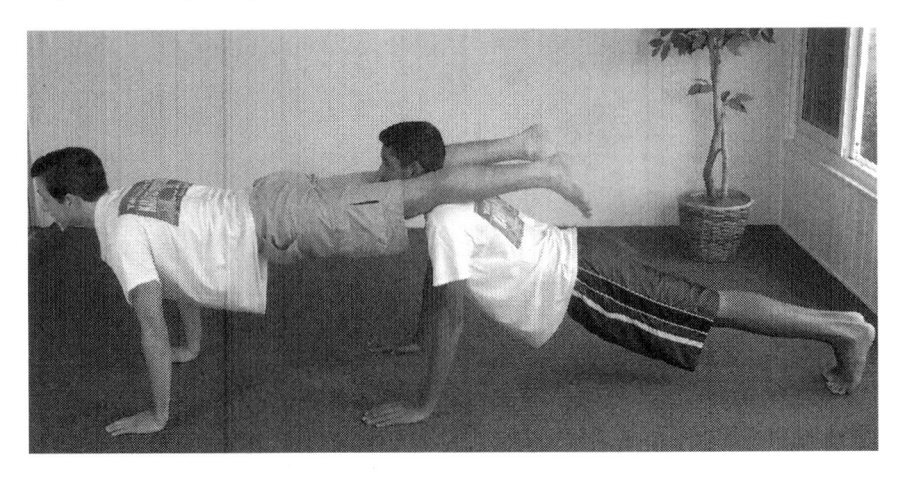

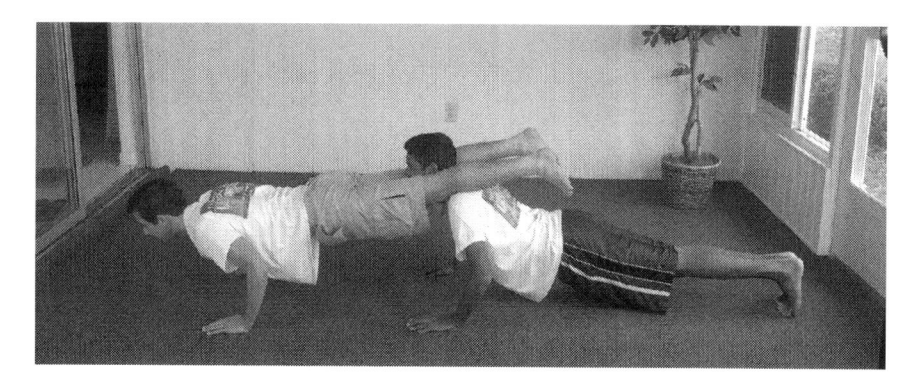

I call these "mountain push-ups." Then switch so your partner is in front and does the push-ups. If you and your partner wish, you <u>both</u> can do push-ups together, simultaneously, for even a greater challenge.

In my martial arts classes, I had an entire line of students in "mountain push-up" position. The entire line of students did push-ups all together as one line. Children particularly loved this challenge, not to mention frequently falling down under the weight of the person's legs in front of them. However, they and the adults also loved the challenge and often succeeded. Try it, if only for fun, if you have more than one partner working out with you. If you do not have a partner, you can use a box, step stool, or any other object which will safely allow you to place your feet above floor level. For even a greater challenge, you can raise your feet higher for more resistance (body weight) on the push-up effort. Caution is important here. The higher you raise your feet, the more caution is needed to avoid your arms collapsing underneath your chest which could cause injury to your face and head.

SIT-UPS

Most people are familiar with sit-ups. Sit-ups are a common strength exercise used to build the core or abdominal muscles. There are a variety of ways to do sit-ups. The most common way includes sitting on the floor, feet placed on the floor with knees bent, arms crossed over the chest or fists placed aside the temples, and allowing your abdominal muscles to raise and lower your upper body. **<u>Be sure to keep your knees bent and pointed up to the ceiling while doing sit-ups.</u>** If you are just beginning to do sit-ups, you can use a furniture prop to brace your feet as you do the lift. You can place your feet under a heavy chair, sofa, or any other heavy object. Make sure that the object you select will not tip over, such as a tall book shelf case might do.

<u>Again, caution is important here. To repeat this caution, if you have no partner, you can gain the same benefits by safely placing your feet under a piece of furniture or under heavier objects. You will want to make sure this object is secure and/or heavy enough to counter the upward lifting force you transfer to it with your feet when doing the sit-up, so that the object does not tip and perhaps fall on you.</u>

You repeat this cycle as many times as you can, and with experience and more strength, you can challenge yourself to do as many as possible.

Traditional Sit-up Exercises - Beginners can use a foot prop

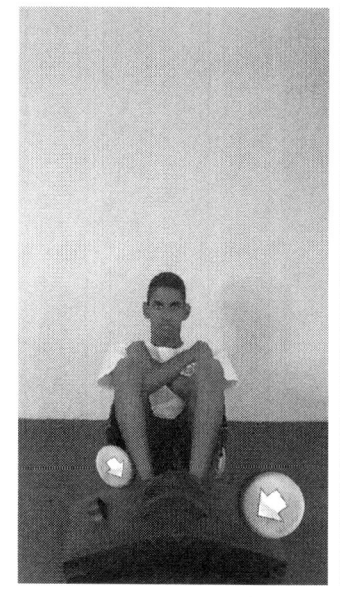

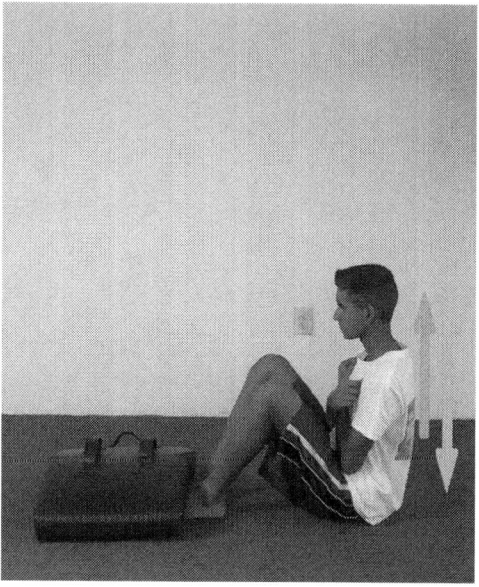

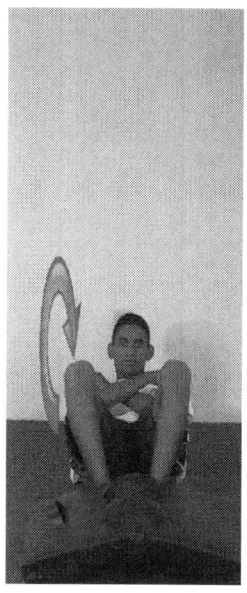

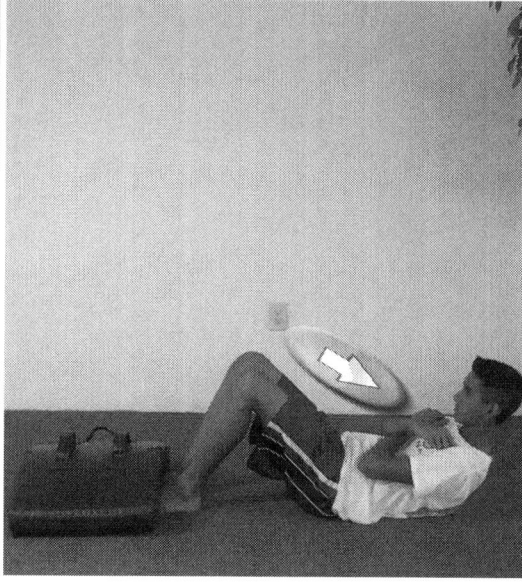

PARTNER SIT-UPS

Partner sit-ups are a helpful and fun way to target the abdominal muscles. Partners face each other and place their feet either inside or outside their partner's feet, "locking" or placing their feet behind their partner's ankles. When doing the sit-up, each partner uses this foot anchor to support the lifting work accomplished by contracting the abdominal muscles when raising or lowering the upper body. Hands should be placed across the chest or fists placed at the temples while completing the exercise. As with the single sit-ups, remember to bend your knees, knees pointing upward toward the ceiling as you "lock in" to your partner's ankles.

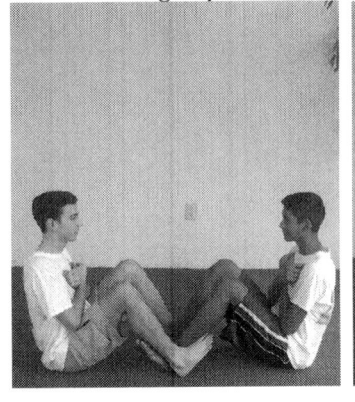

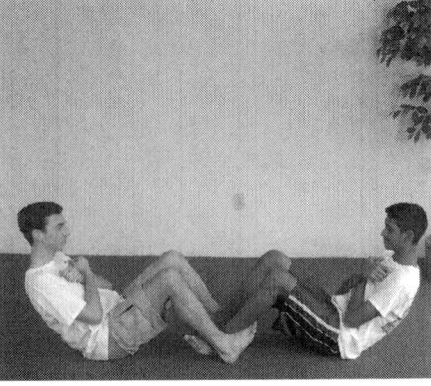

NOTE: The reader should be aware to <u>not grab or pull the neck</u> while doing sit-ups. Pulling on the neck to assist in the upward lift completing the sit-up is **not recommended** because of the undue stress and potential injury which could be delivered to the neck during the lift.

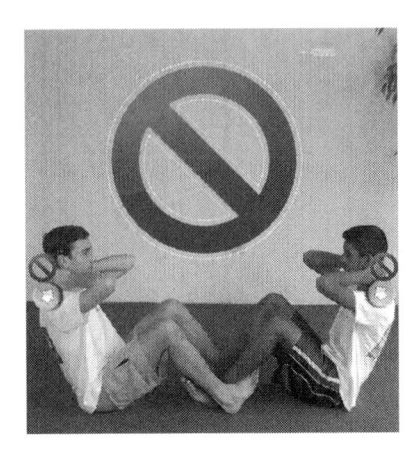

ENDING EXERCISES & CHARTS

To finish your stretching workout today, you will now want to stand on both legs, ankles together. First, lift your left knee to your chest and lower it again to the floor, and repeat with the right knee. Do this movement a couple of times with both legs. Then, standing on your left leg, grab your right knee and bring it slowly to your chest and hold for two or three seconds. Repeat with your left knee, standing on your right leg. Do this knee-hold to your chest a couple of times with each leg.

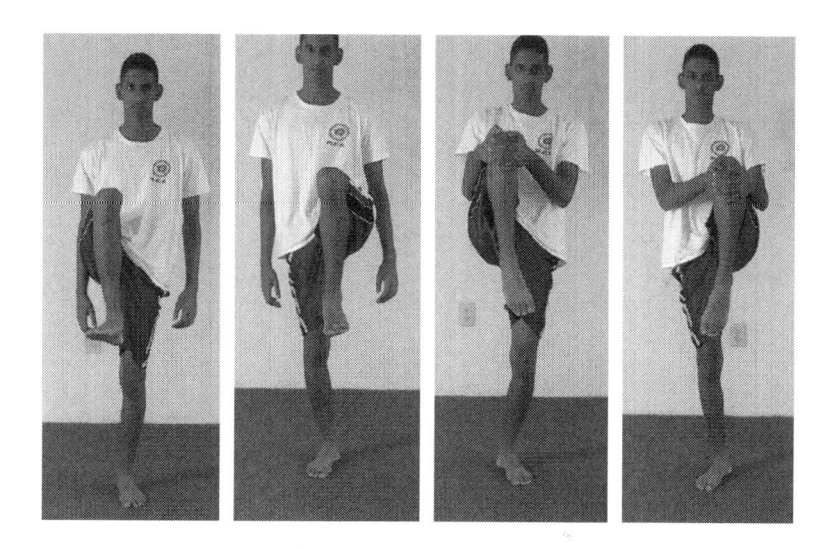

When finished, shake out or lightly kick out each leg to loosen and relax the muscles, tendons and ligaments in that leg.

To end your stretching workout, it is helpful now to do some light aerobic activity to "work out" all those muscles, ligaments and tendons you have stretched. Your first aerobic exercise to end your workout is the jumping jack. You may already be familiar with the jumping jack. If not, it will be explained here. We will also add another challenge to this common activity later on. First we begin by standing with feet together, hands at your sides. Extend both legs out to the side at the same time, jumping as you do so. Simultaneously, extend and swing both arms above your head touching your fingertips together as your legs fully extend, and return to the starting position, arms down and legs together. Repeat this movement about 10 times.

Jumping Jacks

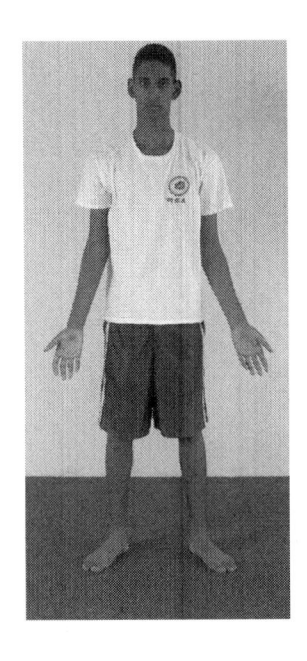

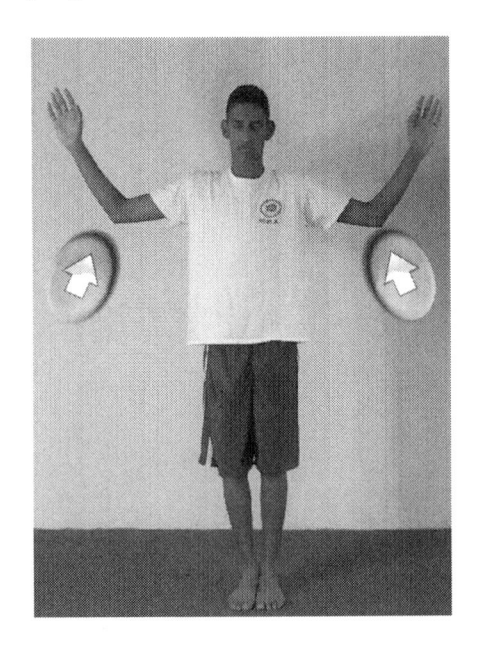

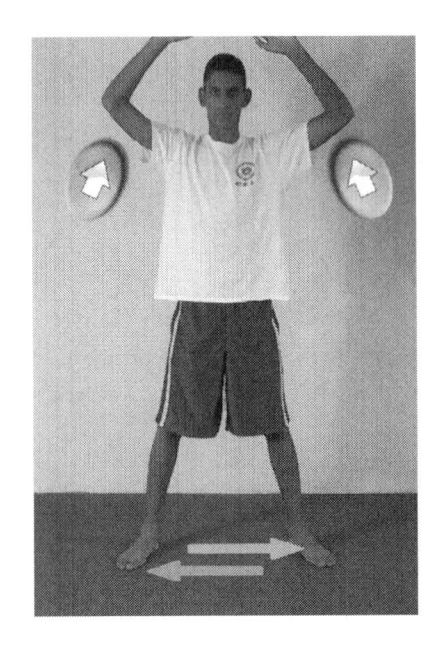

If you want another challenge, continue with the same jumping jack, but move your feet <u>forward and back</u> simultaneously (see below) as your arms swing and return from above your head. You will want to do at least 10 of these movements, as well.

Alternate Jumping Jack - Feet jump <u>Front-to-Back</u>

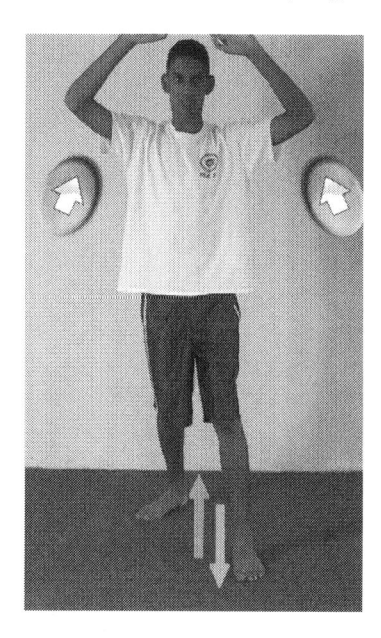

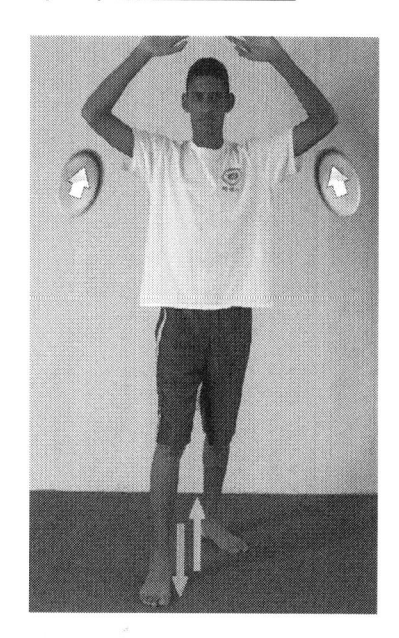

A third challenge (see next page) is to continue with the same jumping jack, but move your feet from <u>side to side</u>, placing first your right foot in front, then your left foot in front, as you continue to jump and swing your arms and return from above your head. Again, try to do at least 10 complete jumps using this technique.

Finally, for the complete challenge, continuing your jumping jacks, **<u>alternate</u>** your **<u>forward and backward</u>** feet movements **<u>and</u>** your **<u>side-to-side</u>** movements as you continue to do the overhead finger touch with each jump. Try to do at least 10 of these jumping jacks. (See next page)

Alternate Jumping Jack -Side to Side, alternating in Front & Back

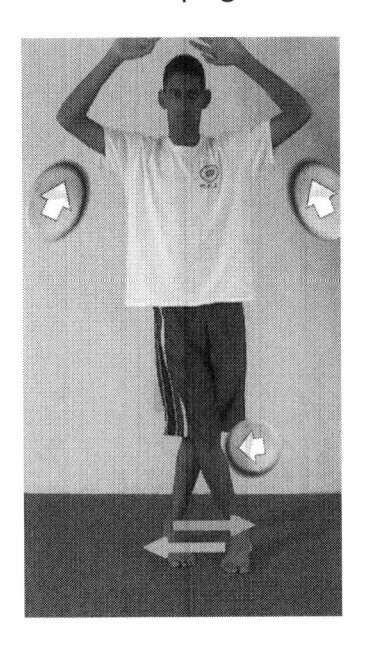

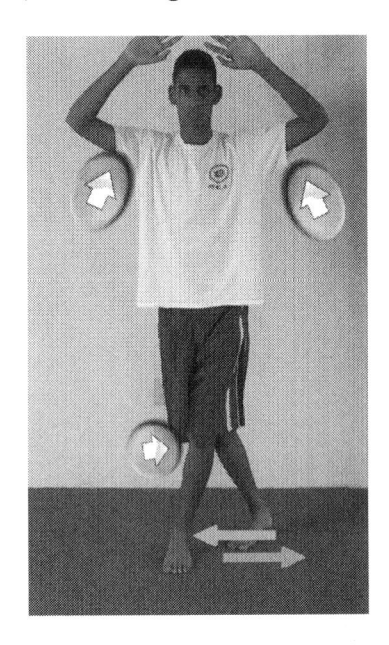

You are now ready for the second ending exercise to "cool-down" your muscles. You will now once again lightly or slowly jog, trot, or run around the room, outside in the weather, or wherever is appropriate and convenient for about 2-3 minutes. To further assist your cool-down, do your slow run in a circle, but face to the inside of the circle, skipping side to side as you complete your circle. After one or two rotations, continue the run but face outside the circle, skipping side to side. For an even more complete exercise, continuing in the same direction look behind you, turn around and run backwards, being careful not to trip. Caution: if you are wearing long pants you will want to be careful not to catch your heel in your pant leg as you step backward. To finish, turn around and complete your run going forward for two or three rotations of your circle or 2-3 minute run. Follow this light run with a quick walk, gradually slowing to a normal walking speed to gradually lower your heart rate. Do this cool-down walk for about 3-4 minutes.

Once you complete your run or fast walk cool down, take your knee and raise it up to your chest and down again to the floor, alternating legs as you do the knee stretch, as you did earlier. As you do this stretch with your knee, first point your toes down as you raise your knee, then point your toes up. Repeat these up and down knee lifts several times. Finally, again raise your right knee and hold it to your chest while balancing on your left leg. Then switch, raising your left knee and holding it to your chest while balancing on your right leg. Hold your knee to your chest for 5-10 seconds, then kick out both legs a few times.

Knee-to-Chest/Toe Stretches - alternate Toe Up and Toe Down

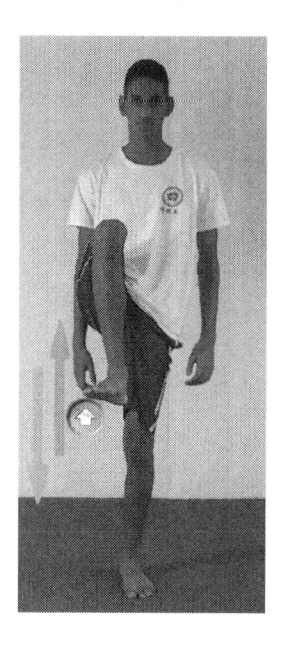

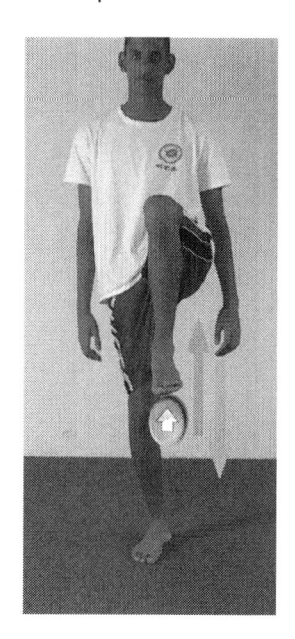

Knee-to-Chest/Toe Stretches - Toe Down, Hold Knee, Foot Balance

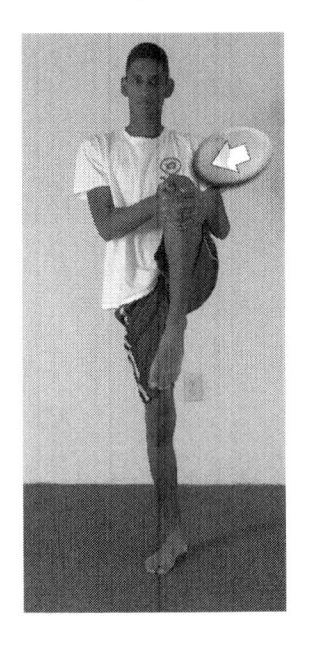

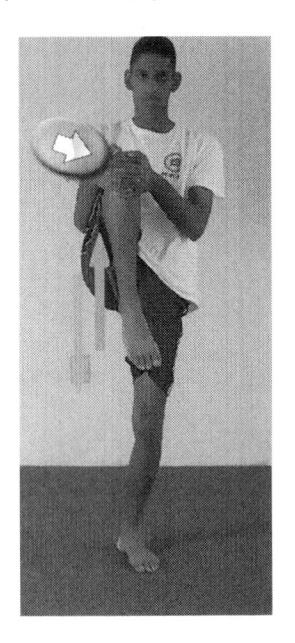

Congratulations! You Did It!

You have just completed your stretching workout for the day.

HAPPY TRAINING

Being faithful to a stretching workout routine will bring many benefits to you, even if you skip a day or two. Ideally, you will want to stretch every day. If you can't complete the entire stretching workout every day, don't worry. You easily and conveniently can pick and choose what stretches you want to do or have time to do. You can group them ideally in the order suggested in this book, or as your situation permits.

You can do most of these stretches almost any time at home to improve your flexibility, moods, and overall health. You can do these stretches while standing, sitting on the floor, watching television, working on your laptop, using your tablet, surfing your phone, having family room conversations, talking on your cell phone, and almost anytime you have a free minute to yourself.

Besides stretching out at home, your stretching workouts can be done during office breaks, at the gym, on vacation, at the pool, in a motel room, in the office restroom, and almost any place where you have a few minutes alone. If you do not have the approximate 45 minutes to do all the stretches in this book at one sitting, you can always pick one or two and do those exercises. You can easily do the standing stretches wherever you cannot sit on the floor (office restroom, etc.), and the sitting stretches where you can comfortable use the floor, such as the family room, lanai, or pool deck at home.

If you are simply reading this book and have not tried any of these stretches, try it, even if you only select a few stretches to start. You can do it. Have fun with these stretches. If you are a beginner, you may need some time for your body to adapt to doing all the stretches.

In the back of this book, I have provided two charts to get you started. **Training Chart #1** provides a list of all the stretches in the book. You can decide and select which ones are best for you. You don't have to all of the stretches, particularly if you are a beginner. **Training Chart #2** is a sample beginners stretching schedule which you can follow until you learn all the stretches and you feel some benefits from your stretching workouts. Try a few stretches and enjoy them. Each stretch takes only a minute or two. You can add more as you desire and your time allows. Get a partner and make it even more fun. If you are consistent, you will reap some rewards in a relatively short period of time. If you stay with it and do the exercises safely, you will reap the rewards of increased flexibility and feel more energetic and strong in your daily activities.

YOU CAN DO IT. START TODAY AND HAVE FUN.

TRAINING CHART #1

You can use this chart below to keep track, by date, of which stretches you do.

STRETCHING EXERCISES	Date	Date	Date	Date	Date	Date	Date
Day of the Week	S	M	T	W	Th	F	S
Standing Stretches							
Trunk (Waist)							
Neck Stretches							
Side Muscle Stretches (Side Bends)							
Shoulder Stretches (Arm Circles)							
Rotator Cuff Stretches							
Oblique Muscle Stretches							
Back & Toe Touching Stretches							
Standing Leg Stretches							
"Down & Back" Stretches							
Floor (Sitting) Leg Stretches							
Trunk (sitting) & Back Stretches							
Partner (Sitting) Stretches							
Push-ups							
Sit-ups							
Ending Exercises: Knee to Chest lifts							
Knee Hold to Chest							
Jumping Jacks							
Slow Jog to Walk							

TRAINING CHART #2

Here is a simple daily and weekly stretching schedule you can use. This schedule shows you when to do the standing and sitting stretches, and the strength exercises of push-up and sit-ups.

	Standing	Sitting	Push-ups	Sit-ups
Monday	X	X	X	X
Tuesday	X		X	
Wednesday		X		X
Thursday	X	X	X	X
Friday	X		X	
Saturday	X	X	X	X
Sunday	**OFF**	**OFF**	**OFF**	**OFF**

ABOUT THE AUTHOR
DENNIS W. BARBEAU

* 5th Degree Master black belt in Tae Kwon Do
* 2nd Degree black belt in Hapkido
* Studied with:
  - Grand Master Dr. Jung Hwan Park (Tae Kwon Do/Hapkido)
  - Tuhon Ray Dionaldo (Kali, Escrima, Arnis, Sikoran)
  - Grand Master Federico T. Lazo (Modern Arnis)
  - Grand Master David Wheaton (Dynamic Circle Hapkido)
  - Master Rick DeAguila (Hapkido, cane, weapons)

Master Barbeau has provided martial arts instruction in elementary schools as an after-school care activity for many years. He has been a martial arts instructor for over 20 years, and was promoted to Master Instructor by 10th Degree Grandmaster Dr. Jung Hwan Park, student of Grandmaster Choi Yong Sul, the Korean founder of Hapkido.

Master Barbeau also has years of successful experience in the fields of Education and Mental Health. He has provided counseling and therapy for adults, children, parents and families in agencies, schools, in private practice, in hospitals, nursing homes, and in community mental health centers in the Midwest and Florida, USA. Here are some of Master Barbeau's professional credentials:

* Earned 2 Masters Degrees including a Master of Arts Degree in Counseling & Counselor Education
* State Licensed Marriage & Family Therapist
* State Licensed Mental Health Counselor
* Counseling Agency Director
* Therapy Clinical Supervisor
* Certified Professional Educator with over 30 years' experience
* Elementary, middle school, high school and college teacher
* Dean of Students
* School Guidance Counselor
* Member: National Board of Certified Counselors
* Past Vice President of the Pinellas Association For Marriage & Family Therapy (affiliate of American Association For Marriage & Family Therapy)
* Professional musician (published composer, drummer, pianist, and soloist)
* Published author, publisher and producer: **Karate Kids Connection-Tae Kwon Do Style** (martial arts books in English & Spanish, & DVD) - Amazon.com
* Hobbies: martial arts, weight lifting, oil painting, biking

www.karatekidsconnection.com

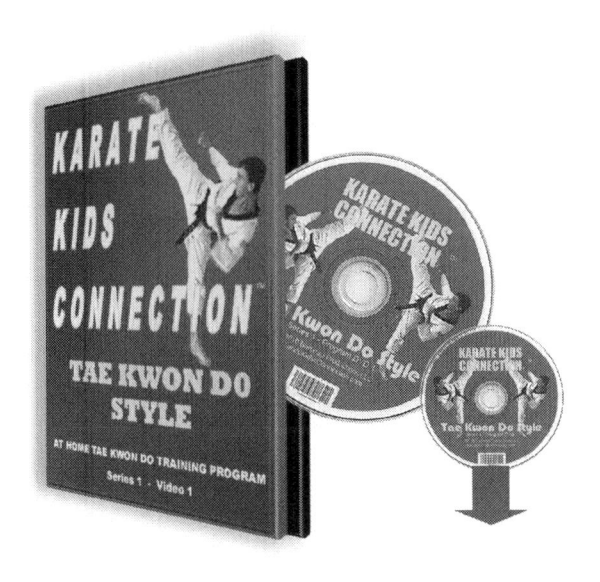

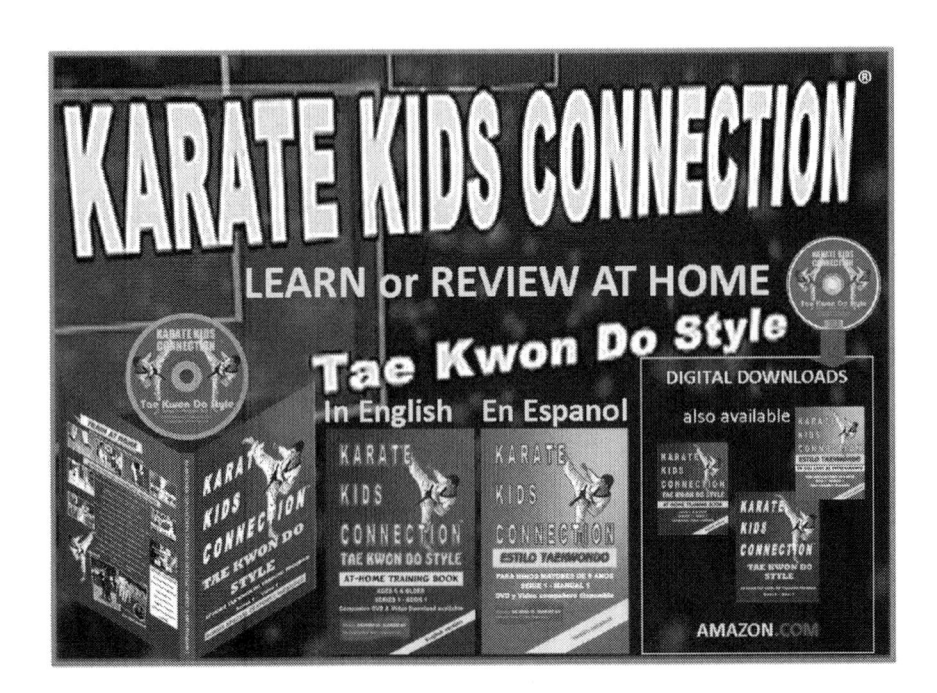

AMAZON.COM

Printed in Great Britain
by Amazon